Also by Stanley Goldfarb, MD

Take Two Aspirin and Call Me By My Pronouns:
Why Turning Doctors into Social Justice Warriors
is Destroying American Medicine

DOING GREAT HARM?

How DEI and Identity Politics Are
Infecting American Healthcare—and
How We Are Fighting Back

STANLEY GOLDFARB, MD

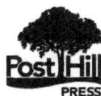

POST HILL
PRESS

A POST HILL PRESS BOOK
ISBN: 979-8-89565-234-3
ISBN (eBook): 979-8-89565-235-0

Doing Great Harm?:
How DEI and Identity Politics Are Infecting American Healthcare—
and How We Are Fighting Back
© 2025 by Do No Harm
All Rights Reserved

Cover design by Jim Villaflores

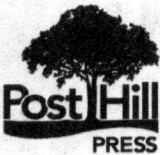

Post Hill Press
New York • Nashville
posthillpress.com

Published in the United States of America
1 2 3 4 5 6 7 8 9 10

To Rayna

TABLE OF CONTENTS

INTRODUCTION

CANCELED...FOR A TWEET

My name is Stanley Goldfarb. After a long and (some might say) distinguished career as a nephrologist, a professor of medicine, and a dean at the University of Pennsylvania's Perelman School of Medicine, I was canceled—not once, but twice. First for an op-ed in the *Wall Street Journal* questioning the effect that DEI (diversity, equity, and inclusion) was having on medical schools and the wider world of medicine, and second for...a tweet.

Yes, a tweet.

In the kidney world version of cancel culture, I was summarily fired in 2022 as nephrology editor of *UpToDate*, a position I had held for seven years. *UpToDate*, the most widely used medical reference, is consulted by tens of thousands of physicians every day, helping them make the best and most timely decisions for patient care. Even as I was fired, *UpToDate*'s leadership team praised my work.

So what was my crime?

I was responding to a new study, one of three that in quick order demonstrated that putting diversity ahead of quality has consequences.[1] I offered an alternative explanation for a phenomenon that had been reported at multiple medical schools. But it turns out that I was questioning a religious dogma, the adherents of which brook no debate, much less dissent. My ordeal provides an object lesson in DEI intolerance of free speech and academic inquiry, especially in medicine.

The article that prompted my tweet that caused my defenestration appeared in the September 2022 issue of *Academic Medicine*, the well-respected trade journal of medical schools.

It looked at minority medical students' readiness for the profession, as judged by clinical evaluations during their post-graduate residencies, when they begin to work directly with patients. The data consisted of 3,600 evaluations of 703 residents by 605 faculty members at six internal medicine residency training programs in the United States: Emory University, Massachusetts General Hospital, University of Alabama at Birmingham, University of California San Francisco, University of Chicago, and University of Louisville.

On average, URIM (so-called "underrepresented in medicine") residents—that is, residents who are neither white nor Asian—scored lower on measures of medical knowledge, medical practice, professionalism, practice-based learning and improvement, and interpersonal and communication skills. (The whole concept of underrepresented in medicine is code for quotas. If race is a social construct, as some leftist intellectuals argue, then what does it matter what socially constructed racial group a doctor belongs to?)

To be clear, many minority students surely excelled, while others brought the average down. But the authors, who perhaps understood that they had a hot potato in their hands, listed just three possible reasons for the disparities they found: "the cumulative effects of a noninclusive

[1]   Stanley Goldfarb, "The Diversity Delusion Comes to Health Care," *Newsweek*, July 19, 2022.

learning environment on trainees, racial bias (conscious or unconscious) in faculty assessment of URiM residents, and structural inequities in assessment measures."

In other words, either the evaluators were racist, the tests were racist, or the training was lousy. Those are your choices. As a distasteful sidelight, almost all of the dozen listed authors were associated with the schools under study, yet they were willing to libel their colleagues as possible racists. They speculated that "in-group favoritism" by male faculty "may play a role in our findings." Nice folks, these.

Now, putting ideology aside—which fewer and fewer academics are capable of doing—the more likely conclusion is that lower standards for medical students leads to worse performance by residents. But such possibilities are equivalent to what George Orwell in *1984* called "thoughtcrime."[2]

I mean, it is within the realm of possibility that these medical faculties are not dominated by racists, their assessment systems are not systemically racist, and those venerable institutions actually welcome minority students. Right?

In response to the authors' woefully inadequate conclusion, I tweeted, "3 possible explanations provided. All are due to external agents. Could it be they were just less good at being residents?"[3]

This perfectly reasonable question, which would occur to anyone who lives outside the woke bubble, was deemed a hanging offense.

Dr. Michael Parmacek, a cardiologist and chair of the Department of Medicine at Penn's Perelman School of Medicine—a man I had considered a friend—fired off an overheated email to students and faculty that read:

> I am writing to address the racist statements made by former Associate Dean and Professor Emeritus Stanley

---

[2]   Robin Klein et al., "Association Between Resident Race and Ethnicity and Clinical Performance Assessment Scores in Graduate Medical Education," *Academic Medicine* 97, no. 9 (September 2022): 1351–1359.

[3]   Stanley Goldfarb, Twitter/X, May 22, 2022.

Goldfarb. I want to acknowledge the deep pain and anger that his sentiments evoke in many of us, and wish to make my own position very clear. The greatest strength of our Department and of Penn Medicine is our diverse faculty, trainees, and staff. We as a Department place the highest emphasis on diversity, equity and inclusion, and recommit ourselves every day to upholding those values. Moreover, providing the best care for our patients means acknowledging that structural racism contributes to inequities and disparities in health outcomes. Only by recognizing this truth, and addressing its root causes, which include the lack of a diverse workforce, will we achieve the aspirations of our noble profession. As physicians, educators, and investigators, we must teach and reinforce this message to our students, patients, mentees, and colleagues. My opinion represents that of our leadership team and, I believe, our colleagues across the Department. Together, we will continue to fight the biases and injustices that erode the health of our nation. Please know that our entire leadership team is here to support you....

"Deep pain"? Oh, please. How anyone could construct what I said as racist is beyond me.

Dr. Parmacek's commination of me had the ring of an anathema pronounced upon a Soviet dissident. It took me aback: Dr. Parmacek and I are members of a dinner club with other senior people from Philadelphia-area medical schools. For the briefest of moments I thought about confronting him—what kind of craven coward denounces a friend for expressing an opinion that any fair-minded person must concede is conceivably true?—but I never said a word. This dinner club is 150 years old and I have no desire to destroy it, or even to introduce an element of unpleasantness into its collegial atmosphere.

My condemner, by the way, has never explained his action, let alone apologized.

This was only the beginning of my cancellation.

Activist students took to social media to warn minority students to avoid Penn. A follow-up email signed by four deans of the medical school asserted that my tweet ran "counter to the anti-racist stance that has been adopted by Penn Medicine and the Penn GME community."[4] My tweet, which was a question that would occur to anyone who had not willfully blinded himself, was unacceptable. I was, by implication, loathsome.

Eric R. Gottlieb, an instructor in medicine at Harvard, disgorged a screed for STAT, an online medical newsletter, that bore the libelous headline "UpToDate has a racism problem. Its name is Dr. Stanley Goldfarb."

Subtle, eh?

Dr. Gottlieb was pleased that Penn's Renal-Electrolyte and Hypertension Division had erased me—its former cochief—from its history web page. I just disappeared from Penn's website. This was a move right out of Stalin's playbook, but anything is fair "when hateful stereotyping and inflammatory rhetoric enter the conversation." Gottlieb never quotes any of this "hateful stereotyping and inflammatory rhetoric"—because there is none—apparently on the assumption that merely making the accusation is enough.

Unpersoning me at Penn wasn't enough to satisfy the censorious Dr. Gottlieb; he also demanded that I be fired from my post as nephrology editor in chief of *UpToDate*. My continued service was "problematic," claimed the buzzword-addicted Gottlieb. No failure of mine in carrying out editorial duties was cited, but I was arraigned for my apparent disbelief in *UpToDate*'s assertion that race is merely a social construct.

---

[4] Jack Crowe, "Upenn Med School Leaders Turn on Former Dean Over 'Racist' Affirmative Action Criticism," *National Review*, June 1, 2022.

The devilish Goldfarb, said Gottlieb, "supports the use of the kidney function race multiplier"—about which more anon—so to the gallows I must go.[5]

Opting for cowardice over courage, the editorial board of *UpToDate* asked me to resign—they even supplied me with a resignation letter—but I hadn't done anything wrong so of course I refused. Nor would I grovel and plead forgiveness for a sin I had not committed. I told them that they would have to fire me. So they did.

UpToDate's leaders could no longer tolerate being associated with someone who, despite upholding the highest standards of professionalism and science, dared to question the ideological takeover of healthcare.

I have lost friendships over my refusal to bend the knee to DEI and the rampant politicization of medicine. In most cases these ruptures were relatively painless breaks with acquaintances intolerant of disagreement, but one in particular really hurt. She was a young woman, chief operating officer of the Penn medical school. She and I were very close friends. I was older and tried to help in various ways, writing letters of recommendation for her and suchlike.

When Penn's letter denouncing me for the "Could it be they were just less good at being residents?" tweet was released, I was shocked and dismayed to find her name among the signatories. I sent her a one-word email: "Really?"

She never replied. And I have never heard from her since. That one hurts.

Since the Twitter blowup, other academic papers have been published with the similar finding that some minority residents are judged by faculty to have performed less well than white and Asian residents. But I'm not holding my breath waiting for an apology.

Since researchers don't seem overly eager to find out whether or not minority students really do perform worse than their white and Asian

---

[5] Eric R. Gottlieb, "UpToDate has a racism problem. Its name is Dr. Stanley Goldfarb," STAT, October 17, 2022.

colleagues, I will speculate that perhaps some of these students are in over their heads. The situation in which they have been placed is simply too much for them, for whatever reason.

Something is going on here but nobody wants to find out what it is. They just assume that these students are being poorly treated and the correction is for whites, and the institutions they are said to run, to purge themselves of their purported racism.

When you start selecting medical students on the basis of skin color rather than grades and accomplishments, you will find that some of them are terrific, some are so-so, and some are subpar. Add in the fact that medical schools rarely flunk anyone and you realize that we are sending some incompetent doctors out into the world. You can easily imagine the consequences—misdiagnoses, preventable deaths, and, for the lawyers, lucrative malpractice suits. (In this as in other fields, those who make the rules don't necessarily live by the rules. As one letter-writer to the *Wall Street Journal* said in a response to an op-ed of mine, "I wonder if those individuals pushing for DEI training in medical school select their doctors, lawyers and financial advisers based on diversity characteristics rather than competency. I'll bet not."[6])

This is not to say that there aren't very high-performing, high-quality minority individuals who are entering these fields. Of course there are. Rather, it says that many education programs and medical schools have sacrificed merit in the name of identity politics. About twenty-two thousand medical students enter medical school annually. But there are more than fifty thousand applicants for positions in medical school each year.[7] This is a zero-sum game. If an unqualified or less-qualified applicant is admitted over a qualified one, that qualified individual may never have the opportunity to become a physician. It is not like

---

[6] Letters, "What Are They Teaching in Medical School?" *Wall Street Journal,* March 25, 2024.

[7] Patrick Boyle, "At medical schools, fewer apply but class sizes grow," AAMCNews, December 12, 2023.

undergraduate years, where individuals have a multitude of options for their education.

The *UpToDate* episode was painful, but I have no regrets. The blowback is coming, in large part because Do No Harm, the organization I founded in 2022, is finding ways to fight and win against the Goliath that is DEI in medicine.

CHAPTER ONE

DO NO HARM IS BORN

Talking Heads asked the question that every author ought to answer: Well, how did I get here? I'll answer that question with regard to myself and, more importantly, Do No Harm.

When my mother died, people came up to me and said, "If she had been my mother, I would have been president of the United States." Quite possibly true, but I think she was satisfied with a nephrologist son.

Mine was the archetypical Jewish mother with a dominant personality. She had a child, a girl, who died in 1930 at five years old from a bad infection, and from that point on she made it her goal in life to have sons who would be physicians. That was all she wanted—and that is what she got. (My brother Herbert was an obstetrician-gynecologist. He's almost ten years older than me, so for all intents and purposes I grew up as an only child, though we're quite close now.)

My father was a quiet man with a very good reputation. He was in the produce business in Lower Manhattan, where the fruit came in and was then shipped out to the grocery stores. He was a fairly observant

Jew; my mother wasn't. But they were both traditional parents, dedicated to their children, and I was fortunate enough to have a very nice childhood.

Neither parent was particularly interested in politics. I think my father was a Republican but I'm not even sure. My parents had lives outside of the Blue-Red bubble, and we were the better for it.

I went to Yeshivah of Flatbush, a Hebrew school in Brooklyn, and then to a rather different school, Poly Prep Country Day School, which despite the word *Country* in its title is a venerable and preppy Brooklyn private school. After Yeshivah of Flatbush, Poly Prep was something of a culture shock, but I loved it. I made good friends, played sports, and then I went off to Princeton, where I majored in English, with romantic poetry as my specialty.

Keats was a favorite. In recent years his famous lines have achieved an especial resonance for me:

> Beauty is truth, truth beauty,—that is all
> Ye know on earth, and all ye need to know.

My love of poetry to the side, I always wanted to be a physician. My mother's wish came true when I earned my MD at the University of Rochester Medical School—a place I enjoyed, grey skies and snow and all. Then it was off to Philadelphia, where I did my residency at the University of Pennsylvania.

As with Rochester, the skies are not always sunny in Philadelphia, but once here, I never left.

I met Rayna, the woman who became my wife, when I was a first-year resident. We had a wonderful marriage. Rayna gloried in great literature and taught English as a department head in various inner-city Philadelphia high schools. They were tough places, but she thrived. She had a great sense of humor and loved her students, though the job was not without its challenges. Rayna said every day was like being in an emergency room.

Sadly, Rayna passed away in 2016.

We had two children: Michael and Rachael, both of whom are happy with their lovely families. I am blessed to be able to see my kids and grandkids almost every other weekend.

For the first decades of my professional life the focus of my work at Penn was research into kidney function. I published over one hundred articles in peer-reviewed medical journals such as the *New England Journal of Medicine* and the *Journal of Clinical Investigation* as well as over 150 invited reviews and commentaries. I also served on the editorial board of important medical journals such as the *Journal of Clinical Investigation*, the *Clinical Journal of the American Society of Nephrology*, and *Diabetes*, and as editor in chief of the journal *nephSAP*, published by the American Society of Nephrology.

I later became interested in health administration and from 1992–1997 I served as chief medical officer of the Graduate Health System in Philadelphia, a seven-hospital system with a one-hundred-thousand-member HMO and a one-hundred-physician primary care network.

Unfortunately, Graduate Health System's finances fell apart and it was eventually absorbed by the Philadelphia Health Care Trust, as is documented in *Governance of Teaching Hospitals*, a book by cardiologist John Kastor that goes into the complex machinations of healthcare in Philadelphia.[8]

I returned to Penn, wiser in the often inscrutable world of healthcare administration. I became chairman of the Department of Medicine at Penn's Perelman School of Medicine for two and a half years and then was appointed associate dean for curriculum, a position in which I spent thirteen years until I was forced out in 2019 for my first violation of modern bureaucratic etiquette. My crime? I publicly criticized my employer for diluting its curriculum, academic standards, and, ultimately, the quality

---

[8]   John A. Kastor, *Governance of Teaching Hospitals* (Baltimore: John Hopkins University Press, 2004).

of healthcare that will be delivered to future patients of the physicians who study and train at Penn.

I believed that the education our students received was not rigorous enough, but since I came into an established and respected enterprise that was not open to major changes, I was satisfied with making improvements at the margins. For instance, I was behind the reform that placed Penn medical students in small teams in an attempt to foster the good working relationships that are essential in the field of medicine.

I was never looking to be a rebel. I have no martyr complex. But nor was I going to shut up when I saw the integrity of Penn's curriculum under attack. By 2017 I was getting ready to retire. I was into my mid-seventies and the end of my career was at hand. I had no regrets, no major projects left undone.

Then I met the newly appointed vice dean for medical education. I'd had an excellent relationship with her predecessor, who was a kidney specialist like me. We had, in a sense, grown up together at Penn. We were good friends and cooperative colleagues. I reported to her and she reported to the dean of the medical school.

The new dean, Suzanne (Suzi) Rose, had a very different orientation. She made no bones about the fact that she believed our curriculum was passé. Since I thought it was quite innovative, conflict was probably inevitable. Penn was the third-ranked medical school. It seemed to me that we shouldn't copy others; they should copy us.

In addition to a medical degree, Suzi Rose had a master's degree in education. (Her mother had been a professor in the education school at Penn.) She told me right off the bat that we didn't know what we were doing. Students, she said, should be much more involved in promoting "social justice." The idea was that to be a good doctor, you need to be a social worker as much as a clinical scientist.

I thought she was dead wrong. In fact, I resented her position. Physicians are supposed to treat illnesses, not diagnose, much less cure, what ails society.

To be fair, this was not a new debate. It had been going on for years, and Dean Rose was merely repeating the views of others who believe that medical education and training should be holistic, not reductionist. They contend that a good doctor must understand the patient's environment: "where he's coming from," to use the 1960s term. That's fine as far as it goes, which isn't very far. In terms of treating a patient's illness, understanding his or her social situation is largely irrelevant. It is far more important to understand disease, diagnosis, and treatment.

Yet the dominant view in today's med schools was expressed by the president and chairman of the council of deans of the Association of American Medical Colleges (AAMC): "A lack of understanding of a patient's social environment can also lead to diagnostic errors, maternal mortality, poor pain management and more."[9]

If there are circumstances that prevent people from obtaining their medicine or getting to the physician, then yes, obviously a doctor needs to know these things. But beyond that, knowing the intricacies of their life and culture doesn't get you very far. In West Philadelphia, where Penn is located, something like 130 languages are spoken. To speak of cultural competency in an environment like that, with a heterogeneous community and a large and varied immigrant population, is ridiculous. No one is going to know 130 languages and the cultural practices and beliefs specific to 130 cultures.

Penn's neighborhood is predominantly black. Those patients come to us because they are sick and want care.

Having the capacity and training to diagnose and successfully treat their illnesses is what makes a good physician, and the cultivation of this capacity is the purpose of a med school curriculum.

Suzi Rose disagreed. The breaking point came when she famously told me that there was "too much science in our curriculum."

---

9   Letters, "Why We Educate for Equity at Medical School," *Wall Street Journal,* April 28, 2022.

I remember—I can never forget—that moment, though I can't recall my response. I was taken aback, that's for sure. Here I was at Penn, which had in the previous ten or fifteen years been *the* leader in medical science in this country. The 2023 Nobel Prize in Physiology or Medicine would be awarded to two Penn professors for work that made possible the COVID-19 vaccine. The incredible new therapy for blood cancers, using cells to fight the cancer, is totally a Penn invention. The Perelman School of Medicine has been an extraordinary scientific enterprise. This, to me, is why students came and still come to Penn. They don't come for mandatory courses about climate change.

Yet the new regime seemed to believe that medical advances and rigorous training of future doctors paled in importance beside advocacy education. They incanted incessantly the once-fine word *diversity*, which was being denatured beyond comprehension, as a kind of talisman to ward off any criticism.

I didn't think diversity, in its buzzword meaning, was a value. We need to treat students as individuals, not as members of larger groups. When you decide to become a doctor, your primary—even only—professional focus is learning this trade, this craft, this science that will enable you to take care of patients. You leave your politics at the hospital door.

The traditional medical school approach, which had been focused on clinical science and aimed at developing medical leaders, was shifting to a far greater emphasis on community involvement and concern for social issues. The rationale for this was the hypothesis that the root cause of disparate healthcare outcomes between minority—particularly black—and majority communities was the result of bias on the part of physicians and healthcare institutions. Only through a dramatic reimagining (to use another annoying buzzword) of the practice of medicine, the hypothesis continued, could these disparities be eliminated.

In many professional fields, academics are divorced from the world of practice and have little influence on the community of practitioners.

For instance, the goings-on in law schools have traditionally had little to do with the actual practice of law. Medicine is quite different. The academic health center is the driving force in local healthcare and has great influence across the nation. American academic medical centers have been the engine of advances in the treatment and cure of diseases. Unlike in Las Vegas, what happens in academic medical centers doesn't stay there but seeps into the larger community.

The event that really precipitated my second career had nothing to do with diversity, equity, and inclusion (DEI) or the gender wars. It began in late 2019, when a faculty member, a respected young man of progressive political bent, proposed that a course in climate change be an aspect of the medical school's new social agenda. I'd been forced by Suzi Rose to attend American Medical Association (AMA) seminars at which the imposition of a socially conscious curriculum was advocated—with nary a dissenting voice being heard—and so I understood the climate change course to be of a piece with this new hyper-ideological regime.

The young faculty member and I got into a real argument. "This is nonsense," I told him. "What do you know about global warming except what you read in the newspaper? That doesn't entitle you to teach it. If you have a degree in atmospheric thermodynamics I'm willing to listen to you; otherwise you don't know any more about climate change than I do, and I'm certainly not going to teach a course in that subject." (I made a mild joke, too—always a mistake when conversing with a zealot: "Would it be so bad if Philadelphia's climate were more like Miami's?")

The argument ended civilly. No punches were thrown, no threats were exchanged. But shortly thereafter came the event that triggered—if I may borrow a woke verb—the ultimate creation of Do No Harm. I read in the *Wall Street Journal* of a movement, backed by the AMA, to teach climate change in medical schools. Mona Sarfaty, director of the Medical Society Consortium on Climate and Health, which claims to represent six hundred thousand doctors, explained to the *Journal*, "This is really the greatest health danger of our century. We must respond and make sure our health professionals are sufficiently educated."[10]

Were Penn to follow suit, we would simply be copying the others. Coming on the heels of the dispute with my colleague, this bothered the hell out of me. So I wrote a letter to the editor of the *Wall Street Journal* saying that such courses, even if well taught, were a waste of time for medical students, for their intent was to turn doctors into advocates for ridding the world of fossil fuels. They are welcome to advocate for this in their spare time, but that is not part of their professional role. (I should note that Do No Harm takes no position on climate change.)

The *Journal's* letter editor, James Taranto, who is now the editorial features editor, saw that I had signed the letter "former Associate Dean for Curriculum," and he asked me to expand it to an op-ed.

I did—and then all hell broke loose, for two reasons.

First was the title that a *Journal* editor slapped on what was really a fairly moderate piece that had nothing whatsoever to do with gender issues: "Take Two Aspirins and Call Me by My Pronouns." That seemed to announce, rather brazenly, that I had taken up arms in the culture wars. I was appalled by this title. It has dogged me ever since, though I was persuaded to use it as the title of my first book. Editors!

The other reason all hell broke loose was the subject matter of my piece. I had no beef with racial or sexual diversity in the classroom—who does?—and I had no objection to a Penn course called "Doctoring," in which students met with faculty weekly in their first year and then less frequently over the next three years. Although the course touched on matters of race and culture, it mostly focused on patient communication issues such as the development of interviewing skills and how to deliver bad news. Actors portrayed patients, so students could learn about these interactions without burdening real patients.

---

[10]   Brianna Abbott, "Medical Schools Are Pushed to Train Doctors for Climate Change," *Wall Street Journal*, August 7, 2019.

But I had been to enough AMA seminars to know what was creeping over the horizon. It didn't take a weatherman to see which way this wind was blowing. Inculcation—indoctrination—was fast upon us.

I took as my jumping-off point in the op-ed a mission statement by the American College of Physicians in which the ACP had made sweeping statements in favor of gun control. I asked why medical schools were shifting their focus from developing doctors who can cure patients to haranguing aspiring doctors with what amounted to Democratic Party talking points.

Essentially, my argument in the *Wall Street Journal* was in the nature of a warning. We want the best and brightest in our medical schools, and patients will be the ultimate losers if we shift the focus from medicine to social issues.

I concluded:

> Curricula will increasingly focus on climate change, social inequities, gun violence, bias and other progressive causes only tangentially related to treating illness. And so will many of your doctors in coming years.

> Meanwhile, oncologists, cardiologists, surgeons and other medical specialists are in short supply. The specialists who are produced must master more crucial material even though less and less of their medical-school education is devoted to basic scientific knowledge. If this country needs more gun control and climate change activists, medical schools are not the right place to produce them.

Then came the deluge. For daring to criticize the spread of social justice in medical curricula, I was roundly condemned by my fellow physicians and medical educators. They took to social media in droves to accuse me of perpetuating racism, white supremacy, and every other evil known to humanity. At first, I thought nothing would come of the attacks, since they were largely contained to Twitter and Facebook. Alas, what happens on social media doesn't stay there.

In short order, over 150 Perelman alumni signed an open letter condemning me. Colleagues of decades no longer spoke to me. When I'd walk by in the halls, conversations would stop. As the old phrase goes, it was enough to give a guy a complex.

Dr. Robert M. McLean, president of the American College of Physicians, huffed and puffed and more or less confirmed my point by boasting to the *Wall Street Journal* that the "ACP has developed physician education resources on health issues such as climate change, firearms injuries, caring for socioeconomically disadvantaged patients and human trafficking. Medical education must train future physicians on these types of public-health issues, as they represent the reality of the world in which they will practice."[11]

In an opinion piece in the *Philadelphia Inquirer*, Dr. McLean's colleague Robert B. Doherty, ACP's senior vice president for governmental affairs and public policy, claimed that "*Not* teaching medical students about such social issues, and *not* advocating to change them, is what should worry all Americans. We need more gun control and climate change activists, and medical schools are precisely the right place to produce them—along with teaching them basic science."[12]

Don't you love how "teaching them basic science" is added almost as an afterthought? It's incidental to the production of gun control and climate change activists—barely worth a mention.

Paul E. Sax, in the *New England Journal of Medicine Journal Watch*, imagined me in an "'OLD MAN YELLS AT CLOUD' internet meme."

---

11   Letters, "Social Justice and Educating our Physicians," *Wall Street Journal*, September 18, 2019.
12   American College of Physicians, "ACP Responds to *WSJ* Commentary on Social Justice Education in Medical School," press release, October 4, 2019.

Apparently I was the Grandpa Simpson of nephrology. Thus was the once-venerable *NEJM* reduced to millennial generation meme-citing.[13]

Progressive students and doctors took to MedTwitter to meet what they dubbed "The Goldfarb Challenge," with scores of doctors and healthcare professionals either boasting of their solicitude for the poor or citing (or fabricating) examples of social-justice issues impinging upon medical care. The tweeter would say something like, "I lectured my patient on the intricacies of kidney function—but he had no medication because he had no insurance and so he died."

I'm not entirely sure what the point was. I am aware that some patients have difficulty obtaining medicine, but neither I nor my critics are going to send them a check or deliver their medicine to them. That is the job of the wonderful social workers who are the unsung heroes of the kidney world. They know how insurance works, what Medicaid will and will not support, and how to navigate that extremely complicated maze. Those who suffer from kidney disease are chronic patients. Many are poor; a disproportionate number are black. They depend upon competent and compassionate social workers. I salute those workers—but I want kidney patients treated by supremely competent nephrologists, not sanctimoniously woke nephrologists with gaps in their education.

During my training we were concerned about the inaccessibility of medical care in poor communities, but for the most part you did your research and took care of patients and that was quite enough.

Advocates for emphasizing the social determinants of health in the medical-school curriculum believe that it will allow physicians to address the root causes of chronic illness in the United States. Their theory holds that poor neighborhoods, gun violence in the community, low rates of voting, and poverty in general produce illness.

---

[13]   Paul E. Sax, "A Former Medical School Dean Invents a False Dichotomy in Curriculum Content, and Advises Physicians to Stay in Their Lane," NEJM Journal Watch, September 15, 2019.

I don't pretend to omniscience. Maybe they have something there. But I suspect the primary causes of poor health outcomes include people not seeking medical care early in the manifestations of illness and not adhering to medical regimens. Whatever the case, it's hard to see what practicing physicians can do about any of these issues. At Penn, I could not understand how I as a doctor could produce better food choices in the community, reduce street violence, make kids attend school, and remedy other societal problems when I'm not a politician and have no control over local city or state budgets. This realization ultimately led me down the path to Do No Harm.

Penn's administration denounced me for that *Wall Street Journal* op-ed with the ferocity of an inquisitorial zealot condemning a heretic. This was bizarre, dispiriting, and infuriating. I had studied, served, taught, and been otherwise involved in life at Penn's medical school since 1969—half a century—and in return I received a public dressing-down.

Dean J. Larry Jameson and Senior Vice Dean Suzi Rose sent a letter to the student body in which they genuflected to the fads of the moment. They wrote:

> Please know that the views expressed by Dr. Goldfarb in this column reflect his personal opinions and do not reflect the values of the Perelman School of Medicine. We deeply value inclusion and diversity as fundamental to effective health care delivery, creativity, discovery, and life-long learning. We are committed to ensuring a rigorous and comprehensive medical education that includes examination of the many social and cultural issues that influence health, from violence within communities to changes in the environment around us.[14]

---

[14]   Sax, "A Former Medical School Dean."

They were setting fire to a strawman. My op-ed had not even mentioned the words "diversity" or "inclusion," and to suggest that I am somehow opposed to "life-long learning" is just plain stupid. This was not a stand-by-your-man moment for the Penn administration.

Suzi Rose called me in and read me the riot act. How dare I go public with this!

"You must be kidding," I replied. "The public deserves to know these things." And that was pretty much the last contact I had with the Penn hierarchy, at least until they denounced me for my 2022 tweet. I believe that their concern was not so much with my heresies as it was with the possibility of activist students causing headaches for the administration.

The firestorm was such that three days later, the *Journal*'s editorial page opined that the uproar at Penn proved that "Stanley Goldfarb knew what he was talking about."

After dissecting the letter from Deans Jameson and Rose as a "case study in progressive correctness," the *Journal* editorialized, "Maybe we should begin to wonder about the quality of the doctors who graduate from Penn. Patients want an accurate diagnosis, not a lecture on social justice or climate change. Thanks to Dr. Goldfarb for having the courage to call out the politicization of medical education that should worry all Americans."[15]

(I was recently gratified when Wesley Yang, a contributing editor to *Esquire*, posted my 2019 *Wall Street Journal* article and commented, "Shouldn't we have listened to him then?" It's tough being Cassandra, the mythic Greek priestess who could predict the future but whom no one believed—but somebody's gotta do it.)

I suppose the typical reaction of someone who is being pilloried and vilified by his home institution and on social media falls somewhere between mortification and outrage, but in all honesty I was titillated. The whole matter was so blown out of proportion as to be ridiculous

---

[15] Editorial Board, "Corrupting Medical Education," *Wall Street Journal*, September 15, 2019.

rather than upsetting. My *Journal* op-ed was anodyne, not incendiary. I've always been thought of as a rather nice, benign sort of person, so to suddenly become the naughty boy who points out that the emperor has no clothes gave me a bit of a *frisson*.

Amid it all, I spoke with countless physicians and medical educators who told me they were terrified to speak up. So I tried to say what they could not, protected by my retirement.

My opposition to the politicization of the Penn medical school launched me into a public role as a critic of the contamination of medicine and medical education by the toxic ideology of diversity, equity, and inclusion—DEI. In time, my new mission gave birth to Do No Harm.

— — — — — —

First, do no harm.

While that famous promise is not part of the original Hippocratic Oath, the pledge taken by new physicians, but rather a phrase drawn from another of Hippocrates's writing, those three words encapsulate a central tenet of medical care.

For more than two millennia, physicians have held themselves to the Hippocratic Oath. That oath, and its enduring command to "help the sick" and avoid "wrong-doing and harm," represent one of the most important ethical principles of Western civilization: all individuals, regardless of race, background, or circumstances, have equal worth and deserve a physician's utmost care.

This pillar, which has guided our society's approach to healthcare for centuries, is cracking. Medical schools now focus on both wellness and wokeness, even as the two contradict one another.

When we started Do No Harm, my initial goal was just to get all this off my chest. I wanted to tell people what was really going on in medicine and medical schools. To put it bluntly, I just couldn't stand the bullshit anymore.

Fortunately, sharper organizational minds than mine, particularly that of Kristina Rasmussen, our incredibly effective executive director, perceived that real change—serious and salutary—was possible. We could tell the truth and expose the hypocrisy and the wrongdoing—but we could do so much more than that.

Kristina Rasmussen is the former chief of staff to Governor Bruce Rauner of Illinois, among other positions. She has been in the trenches of state legislative activities for years, and she is supremely well-versed in the art and science of getting things done politically. Kristina's background helped determine the path Do No Harm would take. She spent her career implementing policies for what she calls the freedom agenda at the state level. This did not preclude federal efforts, but the states are where healthcare and educational policies are really made, and they became our target.

We launched Do No Harm in April 2022, coincident with the publication of my book, which, bowing to the inevitable, we titled *Take Two Aspirin and Call Me By My Pronouns.*

The organization took off immediately. Clearly we were speaking to issues that people cared about and filling a canyonesque gap in the policy world. No one else was taking on DEI in the medical profession. We soon added a second front, involving gender transitions for minors, which has become an issue of extraordinary importance and contentiousness.

We accomplish our mission through education and advocacy about the divisive and discriminatory ideology increasingly embedded within medical education, training, research, practice, and policy.

Do No Harm quickly became an influential voice, especially at the critical state level, where, under America's federalist system, most of the policy decisions affecting medical education, treatment, and practice are made.

Like Lord Vishnu, the Hindu god, Do No Harm is multiarmed. The arm with which I am most intimately involved uses *social and traditional media* to inform the public about ideological threats to medical care and medical education. We have placed over 2,500 individual items in various media outlets, including the *Wall Street Journal*, the *New York Post*, the *Free Press*, *National Review*, and others. As a membership organization, Do No Harm has now attracted over fifteen thousand members, including physicians, nurses, and concerned patients.

Do No Harm's *research* arm consists largely of social science PhDs and other scholars who debunk the harmful myths that have guided the DEI and childhood-gender revolutions.

Our *lobbying* arm works to enact legislation in the fifty states. We're partnering with lawmakers in two dozen states to eliminate DEI policies from medical schools and to uphold the highest standards in admissions and curricula.

We're also on the front lines of the *legislative* fight to protect our children from gender radicals who would encourage them to undergo social, medical, and surgical interventions in the attempt to escape their birth sex. Do No Harm–designed legislation to restrict puberty blockers, cross-sex hormones, and gender surgery for children is front and center of the debate in states across the country.

Do No Harm's *legal* arm fights the good fight in the nation's courtrooms, up to and including the US Supreme Court. We have used state and federal anti-discrimination laws to force institutions ranging from medical schools to hospitals to nonprofits to cease their dangerous experiments in identity politics. (We have found that the media like to write about lawsuits; they have more heft, more presence, than someone merely complaining about something.)

Beneath the banalities and platitudes, DEI *requires* racial and gender discrimination. That's illegal. So we've filed civil rights complaints with over one hundred medical schools for their discriminatory actions. The federal government has opened dozens of investigations, and in response medical schools are abandoning DEI-driven discriminatory practices.

Basically, our mission was and is to eliminate discrimination in medicine. At one point in time, many decades ago, such a mission would have meant ensuring that minority patients actually got healthcare. Today, however, it means something very different. It means restoring meritocracy to the selection of students and faculty of medical schools. It means not creating separate pathways for patients based on skin color. It means protecting physicians from slanderous accusations of racism and bias against minority patients. And it means eliminating all aspects of identity politics from the healthcare system.

Before we go further, a few definitions are in order.

Critical race theory (CRT) is a divisive ideology that attributes all societal problems to racism. It holds that institutions are systemically racist and that individuals are inherently biased, while demanding that society must be fundamentally transformed as a result. It replaces the concept of "equality" with "equity," which means that every racial and gender group should have the exact same social and economic outcomes, even if that requires treating people unequally.

In the context of healthcare, CRT holds that bias on the part of healthcare professionals is to blame for different health outcomes among racial and gender groups. It proposes to remedy this reality by forcing medical professionals to provide different levels of care for different populations. This includes offering and denying treatments, and making potentially life-or-death decisions, on the basis of race. CRT-inspired policies and programs may violate federal law and the United States Constitution. In sum, critical race theory is ultimately making healthcare *more* biased and discriminatory, not less.

Anti-racism—which on its face sounds like a thoroughly admirable position—is closely related to critical race theory. It holds that racial discrimination is praiseworthy and necessary. It seeks to overcome different outcomes among racial and gender groups by actively discriminating in favor of some people and against others. Anti-racism is fundamentally at odds with the American principles of equal treatment under the law and equal justice for all.

The primary popularizer of "anti-racism" is Ibram X. Kendi, author of *How to Be an Antiracist* (2019), who summarized his creed: "The only remedy to past discrimination is present discrimination. The only remedy to present discrimination is future discrimination." (Kendi struck it rich when Boston University hosted his Center for Antiracist Research, which raised a whopping $45 million in its first year of operation. But in 2023, amid credible accusations of gross mismanagement and profligate spending, Kendi laid off a majority—nineteen of thirty-six—of his employees, and elite institutions that had fallen for his routine slowly backed away.[16])

Within healthcare, anti-racism is making race and gender a determining factor in who gets certain medical treatments. That includes the denial of treatments for patients based on their skin color. It is also turning medical students and professionals into political activists by training them to care more about identity politics than tending to individual patients.

Diversity, equity, and inclusion (DEI), which is now deeply embedded in academic institutions, and particularly in medical schools and large healthcare systems, means the opposite of the way those words are defined in standard dictionaries. DEI is an illiberal concept that threatens American medicine because it is discriminatory, it is divisive, and it undermines the meritocratic ideal which our profession has always upheld.

The once-fine word *diversity* is used as cover for rank discrimination. People of goodwill often feel kindly toward the word, thinking that in the medical field it represents a desire to repair the historic injustice whereby members of minority groups, particularly African Americans, were denied the opportunity to become physicians.

16   Sara Weissman, "Fanfare, Then Fallout at Antiracist Research Center Reveals Other Fractures," *Inside Higher Ed*, November 7, 2023.

But in this day and age, when no qualified minority applicant is denied admission to medical school, the diversity movement seeks to increase admissions of minorities to reflect their proportion of the American population. This is a flat-out quota system, which is illegal in the United States as it violates the Civil Rights Act of 1964 and the Fourteenth Amendment to the US Constitution. One might try to create a legal justification for this if it did not require a compromise in the academic achievements of applicants, but it does. In this way, it is part of the reparations movement in American life.

Health equity sounds harmless, but it is actually an attack on core principles that medical practitioners have traditionally observed. Under health equity, medical personnel must evaluate everything through the lens of race or identity rather than using their assessment and analysis skills to promote each particular patient's well-being. This emphasis replaces the clinically based focus on caring for patients with a race-based focus.

Finally, *inclusion*. Such a benign word! Don't we want to include everyone? However, like many words in the progressive lexicon, inclusion in the context of DEI means the opposite of what it used to mean. It means *exclusion* of qualified Asians and whites in admission to medical school, residencies, and wide swaths of the medical field.

Each of these noxious ideologies translates in practice to a racially discriminatory, censorship-happy, and intolerant regime in which the color of one's skin determines one's relative rights, and competence, fairness, and freedom are subordinated to a set of unholy commandments.

Governor Ron DeSantis of Florida redefined the acronym DEI as "discrimination, exclusion, and indoctrination," but a pithier, if mischievous, rival is "Didn't Earn It."

John Tierney, the former star reporter at the *New York Times* and one of our most trenchant social critics, has written, "In the surest sign of its success, 'Didn't Earn It' has been solemnly denounced by DEI executives, progressive pundits, and the left-wing watchdogs at Media

Matters, which was so alarmed that it published a report documenting the phrase's popularity and—inevitably—labeling it 'racist.'"

"Didn't Earn It" is so punchy and effective that at the very least, speculates Tierney, it may "achieve a linguistic triumph." He notes that some "companies and universities have been jettisoning the DEI acronym for departments and job titles, replacing it with terms like 'Wellbeing and Inclusion,' 'Employee Engagement,' 'Student Development,' or 'Access and Opportunity'"—none of which lend themselves to a mellifluous acronym.[17] (Try saying WAI or AAO.)

Still, a rose by any other name would smell as sweet, to borrow a line from a dead white man, and the same is true of less fragrant flowers. DEI—however it is renamed—is corrupting American healthcare, and Do No Harm is determined to end it before it thoroughly destroys medical education, medical practice, and liberty in the United States of America.

Do No Harm is the main player in the US with regard to DEI in medical education and healthcare. On the childhood gender-transition side, we cooperate with other dedicated groups, many led by mothers whose children have been sucked into this world, and who are fighting passionately for these kids in the legislatures, the courts, and the court of public opinion.

In the early days of Do No Harm, nearly every donor and potential donor we approached asked when we were going to take on the horrifying fact that children were being medically and even surgically transitioned to the other—or to another, as some would put it—sex.

I knew very little about the subject, but the more I looked into it the more I saw that it fit with our mission of opposing the intrusion of identity politics into medicine. Gender transition plays into the oppressed/oppressor binary—a word currently in bad odor in Identity Politics Land—and even gives white kids from middle-class homes some

---

[17]   John Tierney, "Didn't Earn It," *City Journal*, June 4, 2024.

victimization street cred. (Well over 90 percent of trans-identifying girls are white.[18])

Unlike DEI in medicine, the issue of childhood gender transition is being covered, effectively, by other groups of concerned citizens. But where Do No Harm makes a truly significant contribution is in writing, lobbying for, and achieving passage of state-level laws that protect gender-confused children from harm.

I should mention here that in the matter of transitioning, Do No Harm focuses solely on children. If an adult wishes to transition, whether through social, chemical, or surgical means, that is his or her business. Government ought not to ban such treatments or surgeries. Whether or not taxpayers should have to foot the bill is a whole other question—but such a permanently life-altering decision cannot be made by a child.

Children simply are not capable of informed consent to radical and irreversible treatments or surgery. Many of those seeking what is euphemistically called "gender-affirming care" display comorbidities including anxiety, depression, autism, suicidal ideation or attempts, self-harm, and borderline personality disorder, among others. They are often deeply troubled kids, and it is our position that they should not receive gender-altering treatments until they reach eighteen years of age. After that, it's up to them.

Do No Harm's position on this comports with the views of the majority of Americans, and our skillful lobbyists have helped secure passage of protective legislation in twenty-five states, with several others on the verge of approval as I write this.

Ultimately, the trans issue may be transitory—in part due to the reforms Do No Harm is helping to enact in states across America.

You see, if we succeed in our lobbying efforts, lawsuits and the possibility thereof will put an end to childhood transitioning. There are already upwards of fifty lawsuits in the works against hospitals,

---

[18] Abigail Shrier, *Irreversible Damage: The Transgender Craze Seducing Our Daughters* (Washington, DC: Regnery Publishing, 2021), 154.

physicians, and pharmaceutical companies by people who regret transitioning, and insurance companies and medical centers will not be able to afford the resultant expense. They will need to put aside money for twenty-five years to cover these costs, because the bills that Do No Harm is supporting have quarter-century windows. So when a fourteen-year-old who undergoes a voluntary mastectomy in 2025 rues that decision in 2047, she will be able to file suit against the medical center, the doctors, the pharmaceutical companies, and whichever other persons or institutions have effected their transition.

We will delve deeper into the childhood gender-transition issue in Chapter Six.

Do No Harm has become the rallying point for doctors, nurses, and other medical personnel who are distressed by the ways that DEI, CRT, and identity politics have distorted our profession and eroded the quality of medical care in the United States. We receive constant encouragement from colleagues who tell us that they are repelled by what is going on. This is no academic exercise: DEI is weakening healthcare—and by extension, health—in our country.

At the most practical level, we have built a legal and legislative infrastructure from which we fight against DEI and identity politics and for a return to competence and integrity in medical schools and the profession.

We don't pontificate; we research, we publish, we litigate, we lobby, and we actively search out young people and aspiring healthcare professionals who are being harmed by DEI zealotry and identity politics.

We have been so successful in this mission that participants in a recent panel discussion at Harvard medical school declared that Do No Harm and I were the biggest problem DEI faces in medical education. If we are troublemakers, I see this as making "good trouble."

Can Do No Harm cure the DEI infection in American medicine? We have to try. The future of healthcare hangs in the balance. So does the health of every American.

CHAPTER TWO

THE MEDICAL PROFESSION ADOPTS DEI—OR IS IT DIE?

As an intern and later a young physician at Penn I was lucky to have excellent role models, both kidney doctors: Arnold "Bud" Relman, a distinguished clinician who became editor of the *New England Journal of Medicine* (I can only imagine what he would think of the *NEJM* in its current, woke-distorted phase); and Sam Thier, who would serve as president of Massachusetts General Hospital and the American Federation of Clinical Research, among many other notable achievements.

Bud Relman was rigid, hard-driving, autocratic—and brilliant. As chairman of the Department of Medicine at Penn, Relman was a transformative presence. He brought in a cadre of young faculty members from Harvard and raised the medical school to another level.

He wasn't well-liked, but he was very influential.

Sam Thier, on the other hand, was adulated by all who came into contact with him. Every young person wanted to be like him. He was demanding but ultra-charismatic, lighting up whichever room he entered.

Relman brought Thier to Penn as his director of the medical residency at a time when that drove academic medicine. The extraordinary advances in imaging have since elevated other fields above internal medicine in terms of prestige, but in that era Sam Thier was the dominant intellectual force in academic medicine's major field. Sam later went to New Haven to serve as chairman of medicine at Yale where, Pied Piper–like, he attracted a new set of accomplished people. Thereafter he taught at Harvard and was instrumental in the merger of Massachusetts General Hospital with Brigham and Women's Hospital, the two great hospitals in Boston.

Unlike Relman, Sam was not a researcher. He succeeded by force of intellect and personality. A lot of very talented men and women became kidney docs and nephrologists because they met Bud Relman and Sam Thier.

A third giant of nephrology and hero of mine was Donald Seldin, one of modern medicine's leading lights, who spoke courageously and prophetically against the politicization of medicine.

Dr. Seldin was a Yale University School of Medicine graduate. A captain in the US Army Medical Corps, he gave expert testimony at the Nuremburg trial of a Nazi physician who had experimented on human subjects at the Dachau death camp. Dr. Seldin returned to teach at Yale after military service, but in 1951 he decamped to Dallas, where he built, more or less from scratch—or at least Quonset huts—what became the University of Texas Southwestern Medical Center, one of the world's greatest medical institutions. It has been home to six Nobel Prize winners.

"The Boundaries of Medicine," Dr. Seldin's 1981 speech to the Association of American Physicians, an august company of senior research physicians, warned against the politicization of medicine. His knowledge of Nazi atrocities committed by men of science convinced him that politics must never intrude upon medicine. The kernel of Dr. Seldin's argument was that "medicine is a very narrow discipline. Its goals may be defined as the relief of pain, the prevention of disability, and the postponement of death by the application of the theoretical knowledge incorporated in medical science to individual patients."[19]

This would seem to be a full enough plate for any calling or profession, but progressives bent on politicizing medicine thought it too narrow and constricting. The purpose of healthcare is to care for patients, not to provide political platforms or social prestige or a healthy bank account for physicians. (I hasten to add that many politically progressive physicians are solidly within the Donald Seldin camp. They believe that agitprop, no matter where on the political spectrum it originates, has no place in healthcare.)

Dr. Seldin's argument, boiled down to its essence, was keep politics out of medicine.

His speech generated controversy, though his stature was such—and the times were different enough from today—that no one threw tomatoes, let alone slurs and slanders, at the eminent Dr. Seldin.

Unfortunately, his view did not prevail. In due course, it was swamped.

In the midst of a global pandemic, as CRT and DEI were running rampant, the death of George Floyd on May 25, 2020, set off a series of violent protests and riots that went far beyond Mr. Floyd's Minneapolis. In a flurry of virtue signaling, multiple institutions set about promoting ill-conceived reforms and policies aimed at installing "racial equity" and identity politics in the worlds of business, culture, and government. In higher education, a domain long influenced by ideas derived from Marxist critical theories about race, gender, environmental "justice," and an overall woke worldview, the protest movement catalyzed a deeper

---

[19]   Victor L. Schuster, "Donald W. Seldin, MD (1920–2018)," *Kidney International* 94, no. 3 (September 2018): 438. See also Stanley Goldfarb, *Take Two Aspirin and Call Me By My Pronouns* (New York: Bombardier Books, 2022), 17–18.

push to implement diversity policies in schools and colleges. Medical schools were no exception to the trend, as medical students who organized under such names as White Coats for Black Lives (WCBL) became more aggressive in demanding that university administrations amp up racialized policies and "anti-racist" trainings in their existing diversity programs.

Virtually every major medical organization—the American Medical Association, the Association of American Medical Colleges, the American College of Physicians, and the American Board of Internal Medicine (ABIM)—went all-in for DEI, the racialization of medicine, and childhood gender transitioning. They adduced no solid evidence for the efficacy or wisdom of any of these enthusiasms, but they are foursquare behind each of them, and they brook no dissent.

These professional societies comprise some of the best minds in their fields, people who have the capability to review the literature and call out the baseless assertions of the DEI crowd, but overwhelmingly these men and women stick their heads in the sand. They are afraid of the mob.

So they genuflect ritualistically whenever the magic trigrammaton DEI is invoked. When the movement came under fire in early 2024, several self-described "leading health care and medical associations from across the country" issued a platitudinous statement in support of the suddenly embattled diversity, equity, and inclusion.

The acronym-clotted monolith—AMA, AAMC, the Accreditation Council for Continuing Medical Education (ACCME), Accreditation Council for Graduate Medical Education (ACGME), American Board of Medical Specialties (ABMS), American Osteopathic Association (AOA), Council of Medical Specialty Societies (CMSS), National Board of Medical Examiners (NBME), National Board of Osteopathic Medical Examiners (NBOME), and the National Resident Matching Program (NRMP)—harrumphed to the world:

> Our efforts to promote diversity, equity, and inclusion (DEI) seek to address the long-standing and well-documented inequities in our healthcare system and its impact on the health of our patients and communities. Excellence in patient care cannot exist until we have a physician workforce capable of caring for our patients and their needs holistically, and until the profession of medicine is accessible to all qualified individuals.[20]

As we shall see, the policies that follow from such pronouncements do *not* conduce to excellence in patient care.

Do No Harm offers an alternative point of view that has been absent in recent years from the AMA, AAMC, and other medical societies and organizations. The ideological conformity of these groups is suffocating; we are a breath of badly needed fresh air. Our papers, reports, and studies challenge the rote platitudes and lifeless clichés disgorged by the woke-captured institutions.

I have come to see that the administrative branch of these organizations is the nub of the problem.

The leadership of medical organizations is rooted in academia. It's changed a bit in recent years, but when I came out of medical school the president of these societies would almost invariably be a well-known researcher, a revered basic scientist who had written seminal papers and won prestigious awards.

Today's organizational presidents are, as a rule, less distinguished. Typically, they have not made significant contributions to the scientific literature of their field. They're no slouches, but seldom are they Donald Seldins.

The management and full-time staff people are the ones generating most of the DEI and gender radicalism to which these organizations

---

20 AMA et al., "Statement on Improving Health Through DEI," press release, March 26, 2024.

have attached themselves. They devise the policy, they arrange the lectures and symposia, they generate the statements, and the leadership, unwilling to be slandered as racist or transphobic by tweet-happy underlings and internet trolls, goes along with it. By the time their eyes are opened to what's going on the revolution is well in place.

Activist members of the AAMC and the ABIM and the kidney societies and all the rest are calling the shots, and they are perfectly willing—even perversely willing—to aim their fire at fellow members who offer even half-hearted dissent.

The AMA is a curious case. It is predictably all-in for DEI and so-called "gender-affirming care," but if you look at its website the dominant theme is economic benefits for physicians. They talk the woke talk but they walk the bank-account walk. Their insurance program is probably the main reason doctors join—it resembles an AARP for MDs in that regard—but even so, the AMA is hemorrhaging members. Once upon a time most American doctors joined the organization, yet the fraction of US physicians who have an AMA membership has plummeted from 75 percent in the 1950s to about 15 percent today.[21] (There are just over one million active physicians in the United States.[22])

It's not quite "go woke, go broke," but it's not exactly thriving.

The AAMC comprises 171 accredited US and Canadian medical schools.[23] It is the governing body of medical schools and the parent of their accrediting agency, the Liaison Committee on Medical Education (LCME), so it is a major tone-setter.

The AAMC, like most other medical organizations, raced headlong into radical politics in the Great Awokening. By June 1st of that *annus horribilis* of 2020, AAMC president David J. Skorton and chief diversity

---

[21]   Roger Collier, "American Medical Association membership woes continue," *Canadian Medical Association Journal* 183, no. 11 (2011): E713.

[22]   Jenny Yang, "Total number of active physicians in the U.S., as of May 2024, by state," Statista, August 6, 2024, https://www.statista.com/statistics/186269/total-active-physicians-in-the-us.

[23]   "About Us," Association of American Medical Colleges, https://www.aamc.org/about-us.

and inclusion officer David A. Acosta issued an unhinged statement that reflected the views of few in that organization other than its politicized vanguard and its cowardly leadership. The "AAMC Statement on Police Brutality and Racism in America and Their Impact on Health" was alternately incendiary and platitudinous. Representative paragraphs include:

> For too long, racism has been an ugly, destructive mark on America's soul. Throughout our country's history, racism has affected every aspect of our collective national life—from education to opportunity, personal safety to community stability, to the health of people in our cities large and small, and in rural America.

> Over the past three months, the coronavirus pandemic has laid bare the racial health inequities harming our Black communities, exposing the structures, systems, and policies that create social and economic conditions that lead to health disparities, poor health outcomes, and lower life expectancy.

> Now, the brutal and shocking deaths of George Floyd, Breonna Taylor, and Ahmaud Arbery have shaken our nation to its core and once again tragically demonstrated the everyday danger of being Black in America. Police brutality is a striking demonstration of the legacy racism has had in our society over decades. This violence has eroded trust of the police within Black and other communities of color who are consistently victims of marginalization, focused oppression, racial profiling, and egregious acts of discrimination.

The laundry list of "bold action[s]" that these comfortable bureaucrats pledged to undertake included a promise to "employ anti-racist and unconscious bias training and engage in interracial dialogues that will dispel the misrepresentations that dehumanize our Black community members and other marginalized groups."[24]

Plumbing the depths of med-school radicalism, the AAMC has even recommended that medical schools offer diversity scorecards similar to the "Racial Justice Report Card" of White Coats for Black Lives. WCBL's report card includes the demand that "Black, Indigenous, and Latinx residents/fellows are [to be] represented in all programs at rates corresponding to the demographics of the US population (13% Black, 1% Indigenous, 17% Latinx)." Never mind, as psychiatrist Sally Satel writes, "that such proportions do not reflect the demographics of the qualified medical school applicant pool."[25] In fact, white males, who make up a little less than 60 percent of the population, now constitute just 56 percent of US physicians.[26] Thus they are underrepresented in medicine—but don't expect the AAMC and its brethren to take up their cause.

In 2022, the AAMC published "Diversity, Equity, and Inclusion Competencies Across the Learning Continuum," which was to serve as the basis for DEI instruction. Seizing upon the coronavirus and the Black Lives Matter protests, the authors declared, "Recent broad societal calls for social justice and the disparate impacts of the COVID-19 pandemic have added urgency to the need for improved integration of diversity, equity, inclusion, and anti-racism in medical education and training." They asserted that "racism and bias" are endemic in American medicine and demanded that medical students be indoctrinated in such DEI commandments as:

— Advocating for a Diverse Health Care Team and System
— Mitigating Stigma and Implicit and Explicit Biases

[24]   David J. Skorton and David A. Acosta, "AAMC Statement on Police Brutality and Racism in America and Their Impact on Health," press release, June 1, 2020.
[25]   Sally Satel, "Physicians, Heal Thyselves," *Commentary*, October 26, 2023.
[26]   "Diversity in Medicine: Facts and Figures 2019," Association of American Medical Colleges, https://www.aamc.org/data-reports/workforce/data/figure-18-percentage-all-active-physicians-race/ethnicity-2018.

— Practicing Anti-racism and Critical Consciousness in Health Care[27]

Nowhere is there acknowledgement that these terms, and the policies they connote, are up for discussion. Hesitate to applaud and you're a thought criminal.

Dr. Darrell Kirch, president of the AAMC, praised the radical White Coats for Black Lives for "sparking dialogue rather than division" with its gimmick of "staging on-campus die-ins." WCBL, whose goals include "national medical school curricular standards" and mandatory courses in "structural racism" and "unconscious racial bias" in medical schools, had a powerful ally at AAMC.[28]

More recently, White Coats for Black Lives, which has chapters at almost half (seventy-five) of US medical schools, has graduated, or degenerated, into apologetics for terrorism, specifically the October 7, 2023, atrocity in which Hamas butchered more than 1,200 men, women, and children in southern Israel. In response, WCBL accused Israel of committing "genocide," with its Minnesota chapter adding that the Palestinians should "free themselves from their oppressors by any means necessary."

Sally Satel, a member of the American Psychiatric Association, expresses a view that is held by many physicians—if stated out loud by few. Referencing the Hamas massacre and the muted response of many medical schools, she writes that a "negligible reaction is fine with me. Professional schools and organizations have no obligation to weigh in on domestic and international tragedies—though in extreme cases, like the butchery in Israel, the impulse to condemn perpetrators of unprovoked attacks might seem irresistible."

---

[27] "Diversity, Equity, and Inclusion Competencies Across the Learning Continuum," Association of American Medical Colleges, July 2022, 2–10.

[28] Devorah Goldman, "The Politicization of the MCAT," *Washington Examiner*, April 9, 2018.

"A better way to use the moral authority of the medical profession," Satel continues, "would be to condemn organizations within its midst that improperly politicize their mission"—such as WCBL.[29]

Medical institutions are under no expectation to say anything about foreign conflicts. Yet the Hamas terrorist attack against Israel exposed some very ugly scabs in American medicine. Some physicians took to social media celebrating the murders. "What a beautiful morning. What a beautiful day," rhapsodized the medical director of a cancer center in Dearborn, Michigan, in an obscene parody of *Oklahoma*, but these isolated and disgusting displays were less instructive than the widespread double standard exhibited by medical schools.

In the weeks after the terrorist attack, Do No Harm charted the official responses of US medical schools to the world's two major conflicts. While 69 of the 152 schools we examined had a statement or article regarding the Russian invasion of Ukraine, only four—a pathetic 3 percent—had posted something with respect to the conflict in Israel. And three of these four, while condemning the Russian invasion, offered equivocal words about Israel.[30]

Relationships between healthcare providers and their patients should transcend politics in the interest of maximizing trust between patient and provider. There is no need for the doctor or patient to know which party the other is registered with or for whom he or she voted in the last presidential election. If anything, such knowledge has the potential to sow distrust on one side or the other.

Identity politics generate suspicion, resentment, and hostility. Once we come to believe that people should be treated according to their group identity rather than their individual merits and that some groups deserve better treatment than others, there is no limit to the bigotry and hatred that can follow.

---

[29] Satel, "Physicians, Heal Thyselves."
[30] "White Coats for Black Lives breaks their silence to demand apologies for terrorist sympathizers," Do No Harm, November 14, 2023.

This is a recipe for rancor—and we had best discard it before it destroys us.

Medical schools and institutions were far from alone in hopping aboard the DEI train, especially during the summer of 2020. Wokeness spread through even the unlikeliest corners of academe. When the physics department at the University of Central Florida—not theretofore known as a hotbed of leftist radicalism—starts issuing statements denouncing "systemic anti-Black racism in policing," you know we've slipped the surly bonds of normality.[31]

The American Board of Internal Medicine also bowed to its activist staff, echoing the words of fashionable activists like Ibram X. Kendi. Its website explains:

> Like many organizations across the United States during the tumultuous summer of 2020, the American Board of Internal Medicine (ABIM) and ABIM Foundation (ABIMF) made a public commitment to explore our role in perpetuating—intentionally or not—racial disparities in health care through our Board's policies and programs. We pledged to move from being "passively non-racist" institutions to being "actively anti-racist" influences in health care.[32]

Do No Harm challenged ABIM with mobile billboards outside its annual meeting in 2022, asking why the internists' organization was committed to discrimination. If it really was "anti-racist," then why was it pushing policies that favored some races over others?

We never got an answer to that question.

As is the case with many of the other medical associations, ABIM has a permanent bureaucracy in place, one that is far woker than its

---

31   Christopher Rufo, "Racism in the Name of 'Anti-Racism,'" *City Journal*, February 15, 2023.
32   "Our Commitment to Diversity & Health Equity," American Board of Internal Medicine, https://www.abim.org/diversity-health-equity.

rank and file. I was secretary to the ABIM's Nephrology Board for eight years and a board member for four years, so I know it well. And I am saddened by its decline.

The American College of Physicians has long tilted leftward, though a former president, Dr. Joseph W. Stubbs, is now a member of Do No Harm.

There's not a lot of politics at the ACP annual meetings, which are often richly educational. The focus is typically on increasing the scope of primary care physicians, enabling them to expand their practices. The ACP's journal, *Annals of Internal Medicine*, is not woke—for the most part.

But the woke virus is aggressive, and no medical institution is impregnable. In 2021, as the Black Lives Matter protests and urban riots and COVID-19 lockdowns and virtue-signaling were near their peak, *Annals of Internal Medicine* published a paper by the ACP's Health and Public Policy Committee titled "A Comprehensive Policy Framework to Understand and Address Disparities and Discrimination in Health and Health Care." The authors, under the imprimatur of the ACP, ascribed racial disparities in healthcare and health outcomes ranging from stroke-related deaths to Type 2 diabetes in children to a variety of factors that included "racism and discrimination." These biases, they asserted, were "both explicit and implicit."

To close these gaps the ACP recommended "actions to achieve…a diverse, equitable, and inclusive physician workforce": that is, the DEI med-school agenda. Straying from the science of internal medicine, the ACP also called for wholesale changes in the criminal justice system to address "racial and ethnic disparities in interactions, sentencing, and incarceration."[33]

---

[33] Josh Serchen et al., "A Comprehensive Policy Framework to Understand and Address Disparities and Discrimination in Health and Health Care: A Policy Paper From the American College of Physicians," *Annals of Internal Medicine* 174, no. 4 (January 12, 2021).

Another 2021 ACP policy paper, "Understanding and Addressing Disparities and Discrimination in Law Enforcement and Criminal Justice Affecting the Health of At-Risk Persons and Populations," advocated a criminal-justice system overhaul that would drastically reduce the number of incarcerated persons. Whatever the merits or demerits of these policies, they are connected to internal medicine using only the most elastic and inexact definitions.[34]

Although DEI ideology had been metastasizing through professional medical organizations for several years, in the mid-2010s it accelerated like the DeLorean in *Back to the Future*, often accompanied by self-flagellation. In 2019, one such association, the American Academy of Psychiatry and the Law (AAPL), published in its house journal a piece examining nearly a decade's worth of AAPL newsletters. Scandalously, the authors found no mentions of the value of diversity in their field!

They *did* find 509 *JAAPL* articles containing references to diversity, but only ten of those articles "addressed the importance of diversity and cultural competency in forensic psychiatry." The authors also pointed to broader indicators of "underrepresentation" of black, "Latinx," Native American, and LGBTQ people in the psychiatric field. The solution? Follow the model of the American Psychiatric Association, which was pursuing a "structural reorganization plan with inclusivity, diversity, and effectiveness as guiding principles." This reorganization featured the incorporation of DEI concepts into the APA's *Diagnostic and Statistical Manual.*[35]

The AAPL may have been responding to the zeitgeist but it was defying the preferences of its members. An October 2022 survey by the group's Membership Engagement, Recruitment, and Retention Task

---

[34] "Understanding and Addressing Disparities and Discrimination in Law Enforcement and Criminal Justice Affecting the Health of At-Risk Persons and Population: A Position Paper of the American College of Physicians," American College of Physicians, 2021.

[35] Barry W. Wall and Elie G. Aoun, "Diversity and Inclusion Within AAPL," *Journal of the American Academy of Psychiatry and the Law* 47, no. 3 (September 2019): 274–277; "White Doctors Need Not Apply to AAPL Scholarship," Do No Harm, May 2, 2024.

Force found that AAPL members were most satisfied with the organization's professional education, networking opportunities, and scholarly activities. Their lowest-ranked of fifteen choices was social-issue advocacy. More than one in five members reported that they had considered ending their association with AAPL, and the top reasons were disagreement with the organization's activities, concerns about politicization, and loss of objectivity in search of advocacy.[36]

Did these survey results spur self-examination by the DEI faction within AAPL? Of course not! They doubled down on the things that members disliked most. The D in DEI most emphatically does *not* stand for Democracy.

In 2024, the AAPL promoted its Charles Dike Scholarship for early-career forensic psychiatrists to attend its annual conference. But the scholarship was not available to all young forensic psychiatrists—only "people of color." No whites need apply. As the AAPL's incoming medical director explained, "concepts of radical inclusion and attention to diversity" remain at the core of AAPL's educational mission.[37]

In the race-obsessed year of 2020, the American Psychoanalytic Association (APsA) created the Holmes Commission, whose task it was to sniff out evidence of racism within the association. It proved to be a task beyond even the abilities of Sherlock Holmes. Three years later, the authors of the commission's report admitted that they hadn't any data to prove systemic racism within this decidedly nonracist group, but that didn't matter: they called for restructuring the entire field of psychoanalysis anyway, asking therapists to "apply an analytic lens to the matters of race, racism, and white supremacy." Ominously, the Holmes Commission urged entities associated with the field to hire a DEI ombudsman—or commissar—to "monitor resistance to change."

---

[36] Ashley VanDercar, MD, JD, et al., "A Bite at the AAPL: Workshop to Help Shape Our Organization," *AAPL Newsletter* 49, no. 1 (Winter 2024): 22.

[37] "White Doctors Need Not Apply to AAPL Scholarship," Do No Harm, May 2, 2024.

That phrase sounds frightening—at least it does to people who prefer freedom of thought over submission to thought control.

When Do No Harm visiting fellow Dr. Lucas A. Klein, a clinical psychologist and adult psychoanalyst, published a pointed takedown of the report's findings on his professional APsA listserv, it set the field ablaze for a few weeks.

"I received a torrent of private support from psychoanalysts throughout the country and throughout the world, and I'm still getting positive responses from analysts," said Dr. Klein. "It's not surprising, but it is sad they felt they had to do so privately."[38]

Discretion remains the better part of valor. Many physicians lament the politicization of medicine, but until the recent uptick in blatant anti-Semitism they didn't see all that much harm in it. They believe that we're giving traditionally disadvantaged groups a leg up. What's wrong with that? The problem is that simply offering a boost to, say, those from an impoverished background is not what DEI is about. Poor whites, for instance, are just as unwelcome to apply for the many "Whites and Asians need not apply" fellowships as are the children of Rockefellers and Gateses.

The National Library of Medicine database includes more than 2,700 recent papers on "racism and medicine." These generally purport to show that physician bias leads to racial disparities in health outcomes. Yet the most commonly cited studies are shoddily designed, ignore such critical factors as the burden of preexisting conditions, or reach predetermined and sensationalized conclusions that aren't supported by reported results. These papers in turn are used to source even more shoddy research. This is a corruption of medical science in service to political ideology.

---

[38] "Dr. Lucas Klein: 'DEI Activists Are Coming for My Profession,'" Do No Harm, March 4, 2024; "Final Report of The Holmes Commission on Racial Equality in American Psychoanalysis," American Psychoanalytic Association, June 19, 2023, https://apsa.org/wp-content/uploads/2024/01/Holmes-Commission-Final-Report-2023-Methodology-Statement-Jan-3-202480.pdf.

Prominent medical journals are complicit in the crusade against medical professionals and the medical profession itself. The *New England Journal of Medicine* touts its "commitment to understanding and combating racism as a public health and human rights crisis," while *Health Affairs* is implementing a strategy to "dismantle racism and increase racial equity" in healthcare. They publish piece after piece calling, explicitly or implicitly, for a fundamental change in the medical profession. They're also bringing race and other nonacademic factors into the peer-review process, threatening the scientific analysis on which physician practice and patient health depend.

Even the *Journal of the American Dental Association* has drifted from a concentration on matters toothy to publish a "steady stream of articles highlighting the need for DEI principles applied to admission of students to dental schools, promotion of dental-school faculty, and placement of dental educators in leadership roles in academic dentistry."[39] No field of medicine, it seems, is immune from this virus.

This prompts a question: Why is the medical field so vulnerable to the woke virus?

A valued colleague argues that one reason is that the medical field has become a hard place to make a career over the past ten to fifteen years. Morale is low, people are leaving, and far too many hours are devoted to paperwork and computer and compliance time. In short, the job has lost its luster and become highly bureaucratic—which is especially tough since most people go into medicine to heal the sick, not act as a bureaucratic functionary. To use a decidedly nonmedical term, it's all a huge buzzkill.

Young medical students and doctors may be especially susceptible to woke BS like "social determinants of health" and "racial concordance" because DEI promoters claim these things imbue the profession with greater meaning. They are cleverly and misleadingly packaged and sold

---

[39] Letters, "What are They Teaching in Medical School?" *Wall Street Journal*, March 25, 2024.

to young people as a way for them to do something good, important, and meaningful in their careers. In reality it's a destructive scam, but it sounds good. After all, they entered the profession to help people and DEI promises to do just that. Wokeness preys upon—it exploits—the kind of people who go into medicine.

– – – – – –

The DEI revolution has dismantled standards for admission to medical school, decreased the quality of medical students, and increased the number of incompetent doctors throughout the land. It has also subjected physicians—especially those in academic medicine—to "diversity statements" and pledges redolent of the loyalty oaths of the McCarthyite 1950s. About half of the nation's colleges and universities require applicants for faculty positions to submit diversity statements; that is, pledges that they will adhere to the rituals and beliefs of the DEI regime. No self-respecting person would abase himself in such a way unless his or her livelihood were at stake—which, alas, it is, and which is why even principled young scholars bend the knee.

For example, applicants for a faculty-position surgical oncologist at the University of California, Davis, were required to submit a "Statement of Contributions to Diversity, Equity, and Inclusion"—but a statement regarding research or teaching was optional. As our late and dear friend Dr. Marilyn Singleton wrote, "I thought the Red Scare-inspired loyalty oaths to root out communists were in history's dustbin. Not true."[40]

Left-of-center professors and professionals like to tell themselves that they'd have resisted McCarthyism. Few really would have. Abigail Thompson, vice president of the American Mathematical Society and chair of the UC Davis Department of Mathematics, is one of those brave few. She wrote recently:

---

[40] Marilyn Singleton, "Advocates for Equality Must Emerge from the Bunker and Speak Up," Do No Harm, May 8, 2024.

In 1950 the Regents of the University of California required all UC faculty to sign a statement asserting that "I am not a member of, nor do I support any party or organization that believes in, advocates, or teaches the overthrow of the United States Government, by force or by any illegal or unconstitutional means"....

Faculty at universities across the country are facing an echo of the loyalty oath, a mandatory "Diversity Statement" for job applicants. The professed purpose is to identify candidates who have the skills and experience to advance institutional diversity and equity goals. In reality it's a political test, and it's a political test with teeth.

What are the teeth? Nearly all University of California campuses require that job applicants submit a "contributions to diversity" statement as a part of their application. The campuses evaluate such statements using rubrics, a detailed scoring system. Several UC programs have used these diversity statements to screen out candidates early in the search process.

Professor Thompson concludes, "Mathematics must be open and welcoming to everyone, to those who have traditionally been excluded, and to those holding unpopular viewpoints. Imposing a political litmus test is not the way to achieve excellence in mathematics or in the university. Not in 1950, and not today."[41]

This is no less true of medicine than mathematics.

People saw what happened in the 1960s and '70s to old-school college deans who resisted the demands of student radicals. Their offices were occupied and ransacked, they were denounced as reactionaries and

---

[41] Abigail Thompson, "A Word From..." *Notices of the American Mathematical Society* 66, no. 11 (December 2019).

worse, and they were herded into ignominious retirement by spineless college administrators.

Half a century hence, those administrators have grown even more invertebrate, and no one wants to be the target of the insane venom spewed on social media.

People are afraid. And scared people are silent people.

In 2024, Harvard's Faculty of Arts and Sciences announced that it was no longer requiring the submission of a diversity and inclusion statement in the hiring process. Law professor Randall Kennedy, an eminent scholar who happens to be black, had earlier written that "By requiring academics to profess—and flaunt—faith in DEI, the proliferation of diversity statements poses a profound challenge to academic freedom." He noted, "It does not take much discernment to see, moreover, that the diversity statement regime leans heavily and tendentiously towards varieties of academic leftism and implicitly discourages candidates who harbor ideologically conservative dispositions."[42]

Harvard's action may seem trivial, but it is not. If not quite a "ding dong, the witch is dead" moment, it signals a reorientation away from Kendi-esque conformity and toward the system of free, open, and honest inquiry upon which academic life should rest. MIT did away with these statements at about the same time as Harvard, and one may hope that the floodgates are now open.

Abolishing DEI in public higher education, as Florida and Texas have done, would be an emphatic endorsement of free speech and free inquiry. This is a particular interest of Do No Harm senior fellow Dr. Tabia Lee, a sociologist who in August 2021 was hired to head the DEI department at Silicon Valley's De Anza College as a tenured faculty member.

---

[42]   Randall L. Kennedy, "Mandatory DEI Statements Are Ideological Pledges of Allegiance. Time to Abandon Them," *The Harvard Crimson*, April 2, 2024.

"As a black woman, I was the perfect person for the job—on paper," says Dr. Lee. But once she started her new role at De Anza, things got ugly.

You see, Dr. Lee was excellent at her job. She treated students as individuals and rejected racial stereotypes. She advocated for diversity and inclusion, not just in the way people look, but also in how they think and what they believe.

After Dr. Lee heard concerns from students about anti-Semitism on campus, she promoted inclusion by hosting Jewish speakers on campus. She was called a "dirty Zionist" for doing so. The school refused to promote the events or issue a condemnation of anti-Semitism.

"I have never encountered a more hostile environment toward the members of any racial, ethnic or religious group," she marveled.

Dr. Lee was told that Jews were "white oppressors" and that she was aiding white supremacy and colonialism. She was accused of "whitesplaining" and not being the "right kind of Black person." She was vilified for refusing to use the woke term "Latinx" instead of "Latinos."[43]

She was told to keep her mouth shut. Then she was fired for unwillingness to accept destructive criticism that was not grounded in any objective facts or reality about her job performance and for her unwillingness to cooperate in the uncritical promotion of so-called anti-racism ideologies.

Dr. Lee says:

> Countless faculty and students on campuses nationwide have told me the DEI ideology encourages antisemitism… Look no further than 'White Coats for Black Lives,' a national group of medical students…. [J]ust days after Hamas murdered Jewish families in their beds, the DEI-driven group proudly declared it has

---

43   Nick Mordowanec, "DEI College Director Fired for Not Being 'Right Kind of Black Person,'" *Newsweek*, July 17, 2023.

'long supported Palestine's struggle for liberation.' How could a Jewish patient ever trust a medical trainee or professional who subscribes to such blatant antisemitic hatred?[44]

When medical practitioners are too scared to think for themselves, patients suffer. When free and open inquiry is run out of medicine, the integrity of the field is lost.

Imagine you are president of a medical society. Your home institution will cut you some slack because the position is so prestigious, but the last thing you want to do is stir things up, lest you find students setting up shop in your office, chanting vulgar slogans at you, and posting slanderous screeds against you on social media. You're cowed, and it's quite understandable. No one but a masochist voluntarily paints a bull's-eye on his own back.

Consider the case of Dr. Anthony R. Gregg, who was president of the American College of Medical Genetics and Genomics (ACMG). Dr. Gregg was on board with the DEI agenda; in the summer of 2020, he declared, "The ACMG vehemently opposes racism and supports all efforts to more fully understand and address the factors that lead not only to disparities in justice, but also those that lead to disparities in health-care delivery and access." But the good doctor made one little slip-up, and if the last several years have taught us nothing else, they have shown us that that the woke do not believe in forgiveness.

Delivering a virtual presidential address during the pandemic, outgoing president Gregg was asked about widening the scope of prenatal genetic testing. Yes, he said, we must get it out to folks of all colors, shapes, and sizes: "The idea is that black people and brown people and yellow people should all be able to see the benefits of next-generation sequencing as it has evolved."

---

[44]   "Dr. Tabia Lee," Do No Harm, https://donoharmmedicine.org/story/dr-tabia-lee.

Uh-oh. "Yellow people" is now considered disparaging toward Asians. The ACMG hierarchs panicked. The incoming president and the CEO called Gregg's sentence "a serious mistake that caused pain and distress for many, including ACMG leadership."

Pain and distress because Dr. Gregg uttered the phrase "yellow people"?

Really? How big a wimp do you have to be to feel "pain and distress" at hearing that outdated term?

Did Dr. Gregg's use of those two words merit a public denunciation by his colleagues? The reaction of most people would be "who cares?" but the story followed the by now depressing script. The ACMG huffed that Dr. Gregg's "remarks do not represent the values of the College." Dr. Gregg resigned the office of immediate past president of ACMG— even though he was, indisputably, the immediate past president of ACMG—and wrote an apologetic letter saying, "My words were not intended to insult any person or harm the reputation of the College. The poor choice of words does not reflect my views towards people of diverse backgrounds and those from any stage or walk of life.

"Let me say to the Board and to College members, I am sorry for the choice of words. Left to speak again, those words would not be used. I am sorry."

Ritual self-abasement was not enough. It never is.[45]

This tempest in a teapot had consequences far beyond the teapot. Dr. Gregg sued ACMG, its new president, and its CEO for "breach of contract, defamation, defamation by implication, false light, and intentional infliction of emotional distress."[46] I've given a deposition as an expert witness in the Gregg case, which is still wending its way through the courts.

---

[45] "Outgoing ACMG President Resigns after Firestorm Over Racial Remarks," *Inside Precision Medicine*, April 21, 2021.

[46] *Gregg v. Am. Coll. of Med. Genetics & Genomics*, February 1, 2023, https://casetext.com/case/gregg-v-am-coll-of-med-genetics-genomics.

Medical wokesters are no more enamored of free speech than they are of forgiveness.

One of Do No Harm's members, Dr. Richard Bosshardt, was ghosted by the American College of Surgeons for speaking out against the ACS's invidious DEI initiatives. As the son of a Brazilian mother and American father, Dr. Bosshardt is all for diversity, but when he saw that this venerable organization was sponsoring talks by Ibram X. Kendi and subordinating excellence and surgeon performance to the false god of diversity, he spoke up—and was told to shut up.

Dr. Bosshardt, an eminent plastic surgeon in Florida, can no longer go on the ACS online discussion forum, "The Communities," and speak to his fellow members. After almost thirty years of membership in ACS, he has been banned for life.

When Dr. Bosshardt called out the American College of Surgeons in 2022, he said it "must choose between surgery and ideology."[47] The ACS made its choice, and it's the wrong one. Surgeons and their patients deserve so much better.

There are true DEI believers in this new generation of physicians, but others roll their eyes at the nonsense and keep quiet.

The degree of wokeness varies by field. My strong impression has been that specialists are less susceptible to the virus than generalists, and surgeons think it's all absurd. Surgeons are doers, action people, and tend to dismiss airy abstractions that run counter to their lived experience.

Silence is generally perceived as golden today, but there are individual cases of resistance to medical DEI, and these can inspire the less bold.

Do No Harm fellow Kevin Williams, professor of cardiovascular sciences and infectious disease expert at the Lewis Katz School of Medicine at Temple University, is one such. At a medical grand rounds, a discussion consisting of the entire department of medicine, Dr. Williams was in the audience for a DEI lecture by a representative from the Association of

---

[47] Dr. Richard Bosshardt, "Critical Race Theory Is Bad Medicine," *Wall Street Journal*, September 14, 2022.

American Medical Colleges. She was laying down the party line on racial concordance—the idea that black patients have better outcomes when treated by black doctors—when Dr. Williams raised his hand.

"If you're an evangelical, should you get an evangelical doctor?" he asked.

The AAMC lecturer was taken aback. How dare this heterodox thinker pipe up! No one had ever contradicted her before!

Dr. Williams did not limit his resistance to this one act. He also provided a model of principled action with respect to racial discrimination in the awarding of research grants.

In 2011, Kevin took a genetic test and discovered that through his father, a distinguished professor of physics at the University of Delaware who had told his family that he was part American Indian, Williams was partially of Bantu descent. His West African lineage is a relatively small part of his genetic heritage, but under the Jim Crow one-drop rule of the old South, which seems to have been revived by the woke in recent years, Kevin qualifies as African American.

This presented him with a dilemma. Dr. Williams planned to submit a grant application to the National Institutes of Health (NIH) for support in his research into treating atherosclerosis in younger people, which he believes "would likely prevent the disease's advance, saving countless dollars in healthcare and lost productivity, and, more important, lives."

The NIH urges applicants "to recruit individuals from diverse backgrounds, including individuals from underrepresented groups for participation in the study team." The implication is obvious: if Kevin checks the African American box, his application will get a leg up on others.

But he refuses to do so. His explanation is as admirable as it is powerful:

> I don't want to elbow a colleague out of the way, especially one who might have a better application. I'd rather

win because my team's application shows the most promise, reflecting decades of work that has helped make this specific NIH initiative possible.

If I refuse to identify myself as African-American, our application is more likely to lose on "diversity" grounds. It's a double wrong. Not only is the system rigged based on nonscientific—and possibly illegal—criteria; it encourages me to join in the rigging.

Truth be told, I made my decision years ago. When my study team files our application, it won't note my West African origins. If we don't get the grant, so be it. I refuse to engage in a moral wrong in pursuit of a moral good—even one as important as saving lives from the leading killer on earth. My father, who struggled against racism to achieve so much on the merits of his own work, would never forgive me for "checking the box" to grab a race-based advantage.

And no matter what happens, I can never forgive the National Institutes of Health for reinjecting racism into medical research.[48]

The simple act of marking the African American box would give his NIH grant application preferential treatment, but Kevin refuses to check it. It offends his integrity; the racial spoils game had nothing to do with research.

The arbitrary, capricious, and unfair nature of these preferences beg questions. If those with African blood qualify for special privileges, why not Indonesians? Azerbaijanis? Polynesians?

---

[48]   Kevin Jon Williams, "Why I'm Saying No to NIH's Racial Preferences," *Wall Street Journal*, March 27, 2024.

In fact, the underrepresentation of whites in American medicine does not seem to be a matter of concern to the nation's DEI officers, to put it mildly.

Students—and their parents—understand the new realities all too well. As a father named Craig Ellis wrote the *Wall Street Journal* in response to a 2022 op-ed of mine:

> My son will sit for "boards" in May, marking the end of his second year of medical school. That examination will be graded pass/fail rather than scored traditionally. He knows this is an effort to permit marginal students to continue their medical education. He is concerned and perhaps even insulted by this because he wants to know where he stands relative to others. This is not racism, it's realism. People of all races are going to suffer unnecessarily because of these misguided policies. But the failures will be buried and the numbers will never be known.[49]

— — — — — —

In 2021, Brigham and Women's Hospital, a teaching hospital of Harvard Medical School, launched a pilot initiative providing "a preferential admission option for Black and Latinx heart failure patients." Amusingly—or disconcertingly—when I pointed this out, the chief and associate chief medical officers of the hospital claimed, "We are not moving toward preferential care for any group."

Does the word *preferential* have two meanings?

This is…well, let us be charitable and say it is dissembling.

In any event, race-based care is a fundamental demand of the activist set.

---

[49] Letters, "Why We Educate for Equity at Medical School," *Wall Street Journal,* April 28, 2022.

The moral arrogance of DEI true believers is astonishing to behold. They regard themselves as superior to the benighted racists who preceded them in medicine, and they are not reluctant to point fingers at their living colleagues.

For instance, the paper that served as the basis for the Brigham and Women's Hospital's preferential treatment for black and Latino heart failure patients, "Identification of Racial Inequities in Access to Specialized Inpatient Heart Failure Care at an Academic Medical Center," was attributed to fifteen authors, all but one of whom was associated with Brigham and Women's. Its subject was the relationship between race and admission to Brigham and Women's cardiology or general medicine service for white, black, and Latino heart failure patients. (Predictably, the authors use "Latinx," in defiance of the preferences of virtually every Latino person outside the higher-education bubble.)

The researchers found that black and Latino heart-failure patients were admitted to the general medicine unit at a higher rate than white patients, while whites were likelier, by a relatively small margin, than black and Latino patients to be admitted to the cardiac unit. That's interesting. Why is it so?

Racism! Or so assert the authors.

"Provider bias against minority patients is pervasive," they write, "and may have been a factor in admission decisions for patients with HF [heart failure] at our institution." After casting racist aspersions on their colleagues, these holier-than-thou researchers recommend "racial equity training for clinicians" and "standardization of care"—that is, a requirement that patients of all races be admitted at the same rate—as possible strategies.

As it turns out, and as is often the case when comparing two populations of patients, the individual characteristics of the patients govern treatment protocols rather than their skin color. In this instance, the black and Latino patients suffered disproportionately from chronic kidney disease and end-stage renal disease. Patients treated with renal replacement therapy using hemodialysis are better off on the general medical unit, where hemodialysis treatments are effective in controlling heart failure and are more easily arranged. White patients, on the other hand, disproportionately had their heart failure due to intrinsic cardiac disease, which requires special procedures only available in the cardiac unit.

The researchers ignored the role of these patient characteristics in the admission decision and instead blamed it on physician bias. They so blindly accepted the oppressor/oppressed binary of critical race theory that critical thinking was out of the question. In fact, they admit in their article that they are viewing this study through the lens of critical race theory!

Rather than focusing on individual patient characteristics, their new paradigm was to focus on skin color, even though this could possibly lead to worse care because of admission to the wrong unit in the hospital.

But they don't give a damn. To them, American racism is the be-all and end-all of health disparities. As they conclude, "By assuming the existence of institutional racism across all American institutions, we can turn from research focused on documenting disparities and inequities to implementation research directed towards correcting them while ensuring that institutions like ours are accountable to the communities they serve."[50]

Evidently we are past the time when research and evidence are necessary to wise policy choices.

Although its medical school and two hospitals constitute perhaps the greatest medical institution in the world, Harvard has not exactly covered itself in glory during this cultural revolution frenzy.

In 2018, the school's leadership took down photos of thirty past department heads and giants of medical history that once graced its

---

[50]   Lauren A. Eberly et al., "Identification of Racial Inequities in Access to Specialized Inpatient Heart Failure Care at an Academic Medical Center," *Circulation: Heart Failure* 12, no. 11 (Fall 2019).

Bornstein Amphitheater because they transmitted the message that "white men are in charge," as one professor explained.

The decisionmaker was Dr. Betsy Nabel, then-president of Brigham and Women's Hospital. "I have watched the faces of individuals as they have come into Bornstein," Nabel told the *Boston Globe*. "I have watched them look at the walls. I read on their faces 'Interesting. But I am not represented here.'"

Mind-reader Nabel apparently believes that non-white and non-male medical students are incapable of appreciating the contributions of those who came before them. This is profoundly insulting to these students, whose imaginations are probably far more capacious than Dr. Nabel guesses.[51]

So Dr. Harvey Cushing, the "father of neurosurgery," and other dead white men who made extraordinary contributions to the field of medicine are judged complicit in the systemic racism that prevented Harvard's faculty of the early twentieth century from being 15 percent black. The monsters!

It would be funny if it weren't so heartbreaking. Dr. Nabel and her ilk have set themselves up as the moral superiors of our forebears, an act of breathtaking hubris.

Who is doing this? Certainly not future Nobel Prize winners. At the classroom level, they are most likely kids who realize they may not be the brightest bulb in the room but they can be the biggest pain in the ass. So they set out to destroy, to erase, the history of medicine. The past means nothing to them. Jenner, Curie, Salk—surely the giants of the past harbored some attitude that is not acceptable by *au courant* standards, and so they must all be thrown into the fire. It's a damn shame—and it enrages me.

---

[51] Elizabeth Harrington, "Harvard Hospital Taking Down Portraits of White Men," *Washington Free Beacon*, June 15, 2018.

If you don't understand where we came from, you cannot understand the significance of new developments. You just keep making the same mistakes over and again.

Meanwhile, at the AAMC, the most recent competencies call for physicians to be trained in identifying "a patient's multiple identities and how each identity may present varied and multiple forms of oppression or privilege." Medical educators are to be "role models" who teach "how systems of power, privilege, and oppression" inform healthcare. Another section focuses on "colonization" and "white supremacy." This is indoctrination, pure—or impure—and simple.

A radical, divisive, and discriminatory ideology has captured the commanding heights of the medical profession. But Americans don't want this in healthcare any more than they do in public safety or education, and physicians will suffer if they are force-fed such extremism. We must call this what it is: dangerous and un-American.[52]

- - - - - -

Perhaps the greatest failure of contemporary medical education and one that feeds into the failure of physicians to appreciate the weaknesses and outright distortions of the studies described in this book is the laughably meager education in biostatistics and epidemiology. More and more, medical literature depends on assessments of large databases to come up with clinical insights. The vast majority of clinicians are simply unprepared to assess the study designs or the statistical analysis that characterize the literature. Most medical schools provide a brief course in very basic statistical analysis and often don't even mention epidemiologic principles. This became obvious during the pandemic, when clinicians encountered epidemiologic data for the first time and were forced to

---

[52] Letters, "The Hostile Ideological Takeover of Medicine," *Wall Street Journal,* May 5, 2022.

accept the interpretation of so-called experts. This led to confusion and outright panic.

The same deficiencies hold for reading the medical literature of clinical studies. Without a strong background enabling one to understand the complex study designs and statistical models that increasingly characterize clinical science, clinicians are left struggling with the information and they are once again forced to defer to the authors, who may have an ideological bias. This leads to groupthink and an absence of critical thinking and assessment.

That said, let's take a deep dive into the facts behind one of the most frequently cited racial disparities in medical outcomes: the maternal mortality rates of black versus white women.

In June 2022, the Biden administration issued "The White House Blueprint for Addressing the Maternal Health Crisis." In her introduction to the report, then-Vice President Kamala Harris noted, "Regardless of income or education level, Black women are three times as likely to die from pregnancy-related complications" than white women. Oprah Winfrey, in her documentary *The Color of Care*, upped the maternal mortality rate for black women to "three to four times" the rate of white women. In fact, the gap is 2.5 times.

This gap, whatever the precise number, is alarming. From such language, one might assume a catastrophic number of deaths. While any death is tragic, the death of a mother, whether directly or indirectly related to pregnancy and occurring during or shortly after childbirth, is a very rare event in the United States. Many of these deaths are associated with preexisting or other unavoidable medical conditions. Moreover, due to an unreliable reporting methodology, many deaths categorized under maternal mortality do not occur at delivery but as much as a year *after* delivery.

The contention that black women are at a serious risk of dying during or after childbirth is a frightening one and may be a great source of worry for black women contemplating pregnancy. But it is important to consider not only comparative risk but absolute risk. The comparative risk of an event between two groups can be quite large, such as the greater maternal mortality rate in black women, but the absolute risk, the risk for each group separately, can be quite small. In 2018, according to one CDC report, 658 women died in the US related to pregnancy, out of some three million births. This gives a death rate of 0.02 percent. While a black death rate of .04 percent is twice the rate, each death represents a very catastrophic but rare event. Black women have been given the notion that entering a hospital to give birth puts them at great risk of dying. This is simply not true. Pregnancy has risks associated with it and some deaths are not preventable, but the risks attributable to poor medical care are responsible for a small fraction of the overall number of deaths.[53]

The easy imputation of racism as the reason for this gap is simply wrong. Hispanic women have a lower maternal mortality rate than white women; does anyone want to seriously claim that US obstetricians favor Hispanic over white women? Propagating the poisonous idea that death rates are inordinately high and due to physician neglect or malice frightens black American women and perpetuates the baseless fear that delivering a baby at hospitals that serve both white and black women is dangerous to black mothers.

The corporate media, which often act as stenographers for the DEI industry, repeated Vice President Harris's claims and the Biden administration's policy prescriptions without an ounce of skepticism. *Philadelphia Inquirer* reporter Layla Jones wrote, "We know that Black women are three to four times more likely to die due to pregnancy-related causes than white, Asian, or Latinx women…. [C]learly race plays a part in pregnancy and birthing. And when we say race, we really mean the results of systemic racism."[54]

---

53   Donna L. Hoyert, PhD, and Arialdi M. Miniño, MPH, "Maternal Mortality in the United States: Changes in Coding, Publication, and Data Release, 2018," *National Vital Statistics Reports* 69, no. 2 (January 30, 2020): 1–18.
54   Layla A. Jones, "When the Water Breaks," *Philadelphia Inquirer*, July 12, 2022.

Most media stories on healthcare disparities begin with the historical wrongs perpetrated against the black community, even back to the time of slavery. The authors then immediately shift to anecdotes, either their own or those of their acquaintances. These tales of unpleasant encounters with the healthcare system are held up as modern examples of discrimination, but all types of patients encounter harried nurses and physicians, and frustration with personal services received in the hospital are often misinterpreted as indifference to patient well-being. Patients complain about everything, sometimes with cause. "Nobody answered the call when I rang the nurses." Well, hospitals are chaotic. The nurses or aides may have more pressing matters to attend to. Or maybe someone is on break. Whatever. But to blame every such instance on medical racism is outrageous.

Other stories in this genre focus on medical errors, attributing them to racism and discrimination but rarely are these anything but examples of poor training or deficient clinical judgment.

The facts, shorn of ideological embellishment, give a much clearer and more nuanced picture of the maternal mortality issue:

— A detailed study performed by the CDC in 2018 found that many deaths are erroneously recorded as occurring related to pregnancy. Only 31 percent of deaths occurring within a year of pregnancy were related to complications of pregnancy while the rest were due to unrelated medical conditions or trauma.

— Of the deaths related to pregnancy, 42 percent were considered by an expert panel to not be preventable. These include medical conditions like cardiovascular disease and pulmonary embolism. Of the preventable deaths, about a third were due to actions attributable to the medical staff caring for the patient.

— A review of this study and the national statistics show that a preventable death in pregnancy is a very rare event and that the majority of women who die due to a condition related to pregnancy are white women.

— The cause of the higher maternal death rate in black women is due to high rates of pulmonary embolism and a rare condition called peripartum cardiomyopathy, a form of severe heart failure with a probable immunologic origin. Neither is likely to be amenable to systematic interventions. A study published in the *Journal of the American College of Cardiology* found that African American ethnicity remained a significant risk factor (thirty times greater risk in black versus white women) for peripartum cardiomyopathy when other risk factors were considered in multivariable analyses.[55]

— There are also certain genetic and biologic characteristics shared by some black women experiencing complicated pregnancies. Many clinical disorders, such as chronic kidney disease and hypertension, afflict black patients at very high rates, and they have a substantial genetic component that contribute to disparities in maternal morbidity and mortality. A national consortium of investigators examined a known genetic factor for hypertension and kidney disease in black patients, a mutation in the gene APOL1. They found that a particular form of the mutation, in which two copies of the gene are found in the fetus, conveys a two-fold greater risk for preeclampsia, likely by adversely affecting the function of the placenta. Preeclampsia and eclampsia are leading causes of maternal morbidity and mortality.[56]

— Morbidity in pregnancy is also more common in black women and is likely attributable to the quality of the hospital where

---

[55] Mindy B. Gentry et al., "African-American Women Have a Higher Risk for Developing Peripartum Cardiomyopathy," *Journal of the American College of Cardiology* 55, no. 7 (2010): 654–659.

[56] Kimberly J. Reidy et al., "Genetic risk of *APOL1* and kidney disease in children and young adults of African ancestry," *Current Opinion in Pediatrics* 30, no. 2 (April 2018): 252–259.

black women deliver their infants and to poor access or usage of prenatal care.

The good news is that an improvement in US maternal mortality rates is possible with better hospital training programs and greater use of prenatal care. Better health literacy should be a feature of high-school education. Better access to healthcare is the key to improving this component of the disparity in maternal morbidity and perhaps in maternal mortality as well. The solution is more doctors, not just doctors of a specific creed or race.

Yet with dreary predictability, the Biden administration called for implicit bias training of physicians to improve maternal patient outcomes—even though programs aimed at supposed physician bias have no evidence to support their use.

Dr. Elizabeth Howell has studied the problem of in-hospital maternal morbidity during delivery in New York City. Howell found that black women tended to deliver their babies at hospitals that serve mostly black women. Further, they had more morbid complications than white women who delivered at hospitals that serve mostly white women. She speculated that if black women delivered at the same hospitals as white women, their complication rates would fall by 50 percent. Moreover, when white women delivered at hospitals that serve mostly black women, their complications rate was the same as that of black women. The implication here is that an effort to reduce the rate of complications of delivery and, presumably, even the remote risk of maternal mortality, requires improving hospital quality. This means better training in responding to complications such as acute hemorrhage, or treating the complex conditions of eclampsia and preeclampsia, hypertensive conditions which can be lethal. It does not mean sending physicians to implicit bias training, which, as we will see in Chapter Five, is an ineffectual solution to a dubious problem that only frustrates and demoralizes physicians.[57]

Minority communities do not need different healthcare; they need *more* healthcare.

Bending, folding, spindling, and mutilating data to fit into the procrustean bed of the DEI narrative is distressingly common among medical journals today. To pick an example from a very weedy field, in 2022, a paper ominously titled "Structural racism is a mediator of disparities in acute myeloid leukemia outcomes" appeared in the prestigious medical journal *Blood*.[58]

The tipoff was in the title. In the not-so-distant past, medical articles bore plainly descriptive, if decidedly unprovocative, titles. They merely described the study. This one could have been called "Mediators of outcome in Acute Myeloid Leukemia." But that is neutral and boring and would not have attracted the same attention—nor would it have advertised the virtue-signaling bias of the authors.

Those authors, who number more than twenty, examined the outcome of leukemia patients from six Chicago-area cancer centers between 2012 and 2018. They found that black patients had a 50 percent greater risk of dying over a three-year period than white patients. Since black patients lived in poorer neighborhoods (as determined by census information), and because the authors defined racism as living in poor neighborhoods, they concluded that "structural racism" explained "a substantial proportion" of the disparate outcomes. Hence the title.

But there is so much left unsaid in the study. Whenever one compares patient outcomes based on skin color, the question must be asked

57 Elizabeth A. Howell, "Reducing Disparities in Severe Maternal Morbidity and Mortality," *Clinical Obstetrics and Gynecology* 61, no. 2 (June 2018): 387–399; Stanley Goldfarb, "Maternal Mortality in the U.S.—Media Narratives and Reality," Do No Harm, November 17, 2022.

58 Ivy Elizabeth Abraham et al., "Structural racism is a mediator of disparities in acute myeloid leukemia outcomes," *Blood* 139, no. 14 (2022): 2212–2226.

whether other characteristics could have influenced the outcome. In this case, the answer is a resounding yes. Fifty percent of black patients developed leukemia after receiving chemotherapy for a previous malignancy. For white patients, the number was 30 percent. Moreover, when the genetic characteristics of the leukemic cells were examined, the black patients had a higher frequency of genetic markers known to result in poor outcomes.

Thus the authors were comparing two very different groups of patients, even beyond the patients' race.

The authors of the *Blood* study dismissed the leukemia characteristics as unimportant, in defiance of all we know about the subject, including the discovery by Lene Sofie Granfeldt Østgård et al., described in the *Journal of Clinical Oncology*, that "we find tAML (post-chemotherapy leukemia) to be independently associated with increased risk of death."[59]

It was necessary for the authors of the *Blood* study to ignore this in making their ideologically driven claim.

We will improve the outcomes of black patients with leukemia by relying on sound scientific and medical analysis, not unscientific and politicized claims. The real solution is more effective clinical therapeutics applied to each individual patient. Sensationalized studies such as this one do not advance the standard of medical care. All they do is advance a divisive ideology that sees racism discoloring every aspect of American life.

The idea that any disparity in outcomes between the black community and other communities must be due to racism, which then gets defined as anything that produces a disparity between blacks and others, is profoundly harmful.

Indeed, during the COVID-19 pandemic, the New York State Department of Health devised algorithms that determined who would

---

[59] Lene Sofie Granfeldt Østgård, "Epidemiology and Clinical Significance of Secondary and Therapy-Related Acute Myeloid Leukemia: A National Population-Based Cohort Study," *Journal of Clinical Oncology* 33, no. 31 (2015): 3641–3649.

get the monoclonal antibodies and antiviral pills when they became available. Priority was given to those who had "a medical condition or other factors that increase their risk for severe illness." Due to "long-standing systemic health and social inequities," according to the Department of Health, "non-white race or Hispanic/Latino ethnicity should be considered a risk factor."[60]

If you were non-white, you received extra points solely for that fact. So if two people were equally ill or susceptible, the person of color would get it over the person of pallor. This racism is so egregious as to beggar belief, but it's part and rotten parcel of DEI.

Sometimes it seems as if there is no outer limit of woke absurdity that cannot be exceeded by the rabid. In 2024, for instance, the Oregon Medical Board proposed the inclusion of "microaggressions" under the category of "unprofessional misconduct" for which a physician can be penalized all the way up to the loss of one's license. Failing to report a microaggression by a colleague would also result in a penalty.

What, you ask, is a microaggression? Columbia professor Derald Wing Sue, whom the Oregon state government lauds as a "microaggressions expert," says that saying any of the following constitutes microaggressing:

— "America is the land of opportunity."
— "I believe the most qualified person should get the job."
— "America is a melting pot."
— "There is only one race, the human race."[61]

Under this proposal, a doctor saying any one of these things, or a thousand other seemingly benign statements, could have lost his or her license to practice medicine in Oregon.

---

[60] Houston Keene, "New York says it will prioritize non-White people in distributing low supply of COVID-19 treatments," Fox News, December 31, 2021.

[61] Peter Hasson, "Oregon Doctors Could Soon Lose Their Licenses for 'Microaggressions' Under Proposed Medical Board Rule," *Washington Free Beacon*, June 18, 2024.

This is insane—and I fully realize that by saying this I would be microaggressing in Oregon.

Such a rule would have consequences for patients as well as doctors. Physicians need to be able to speak frankly and honestly with their patients. If they believe that they can be sanctioned because they deliver bad news or make a comment that the patient misinterprets, this will have a chilling effect on speech and ultimately lead to deterioration in the patient-physician relationship. We will go down a disastrous path that leads to even further declines in the quality of delivered healthcare.

When this came under discussion, I could not imagine that the physicians in Oregon would tolerate such a ridiculous proposal. Their protests have resulted in its softening, but its advocates aren't going away any time soon.

Just when you think DEI can't get any crazier...it gets crazier.

CHAPTER THREE

MED SCHOOL MADNESS

Medical schools increasingly are preparing physicians for social activism at the expense of medical science. Such student groups as White Coats for Black Lives demand that administrators reframe curricula around reparations for slavery, decarceration of prisoners, and other topics with no bearing on training doctors to care for individual patients. Courses in biochemistry and pharmacology give way to leftist indoctrination. Medical schools and residencies are lowering admissions standards. The result will be fewer talented physicians providing high-quality care to fewer patients.

Does anyone outside of the most perfervid DEI ideologues desire that outcome?

These policies and practices have no justification. There's no credible evidence that physicians are racist or that minority patients will benefit if healthcare is built on a race-based foundation. Common sense says that patients of all colors will suffer. The public's trust in medical institutions, which fell sharply during the pandemic, will fall further and take patient health with it.

Having talked with many physicians, I know that unwarranted accusations of racism are contributing to physician burnout and early retirement, making it harder for patients to receive care, especially in vulnerable communities. Such accusations also sow profound distrust in the treatment room, eroding the doctor-patient relationship that's crucial to better health outcomes. As race-based ideology dominates ever more of medical research and education, nonscientific factors will increasingly determine what treatments patients receive.

Healthcare is close to a tipping point, but I'm confident a majority of physicians oppose what's happening to our profession. Many fear speaking out, lest the social-justice mob destroy their careers, but the woke takeover of healthcare will do that anyway.

We have to stand and fight—and that fight begins in the medical schools.

Medical schools are a different world than the medical societies, though there is a strong interaction between them. The societies are, for the most part, headed by academicians who oscillate between them and the schools. Ideas cross-pollinate, flowing back and forth, but there are issues unique to each.

Today a master's degree in education is often what it takes to qualify for key administrative roles on medical-school faculties. The zeitgeist of sociology and social work have become the driving force in medical education, and it has suffered accordingly.

The traditional American model of medical training, which has been emulated around the world, emphasized a scientific approach to treatment and subjected students to rigorous classroom instruction. Students didn't encounter patients until they had some fundamental knowledge of disease processes and knew how to interpret symptoms. They were expected to appreciate medical advances and be able to incorporate them into their eventual fields of practice. Medical education was demanding and occasionally led to student failure, but it produced a technically proficient and responsible physician corps for the US.

Unlike in most fields, the direction of medicine is pushed by its academic realm. And in the early twenty-first century, a critical mass of progressive academics decided that we needed more black doctors, and they determined to alter institutions and their rules to achieve that result. There was no empirical basis for believing that the racial makeup of the nation's physicians had anything to do with health outcomes, but these were true believers. The formerly useful word *diversity* became their mantra.

After George Floyd was killed in May 2020 the whole thing blew up. DEI and so-called "social justice" became central facets of medical education, and they remain so to this day. Medical school classes were treated like kindergarteners, as if they had never seen human beings different from them. Many of these med students were in their mid-twenties; they'd been out in the world, worked in business, met people from a wide variety of backgrounds, and here they were being infantilized. It was condescending and insulting, and the old ideal of "let's pick the people with the greatest aptitude to be good doctors" went out the window and into the trash can marked "Racist."

- - - - - -

Part of the justification for affirmative action at medical schools is that if students can pass minimal competency tests, like licensure exams, then they are qualified to be physicians. Therefore, seeking out the best and the brightest who have been particularly successful in their academic pursuits is really not necessary to produce adequate healthcare. But this is not what patients expect. No matter their racial background, patients expect and should receive the highest possible quality of care.

Academic achievement by physicians is an ingredient in creating a highly effective physician workforce. I maintain that medicine is a highly academic pursuit. The way we have tested—and should still test—students' knowledge is through multiple-choice questions on exams. In this model, there is a stem, a short statement about a particular patient or a particular medical condition, and then a series of five distractors or possible explanations as to the origin of the clinical problem. Their job is to pick out the right answer. When they enter the clinics and begin to see patients, they will be constructing the multiple-choice question. They will gather the information required for the stem or description of the problem. They will then produce four or five alternative possibilities to explain the problem and pick the right one to properly care for the patient.

This is an academic process. It requires learning and retaining much information about illness and about the variability of human response to it and it requires judgment fortified by a strong understanding of the basic principles underlying the clinical problems they encounter. This activity requires a nimble mind and the commitment to learn a vast amount of information to deal with patient problems in real time while in the presence of the patient. There is no time to retire to the library to learn about the patient's problem.

Once you start taking in people who struggle to do the work, you are faced with a choice: either you flunk them or you make things easier. The third option—coaching them up—is obviously superior to the other two, but that is much harder to do, and if a student just isn't up to the task no amount of coaching and encouragement will make him or her a competent physician.

I don't want to sound like the old man sitting on his porch growling about how much better things were when he was young, but...

The changes at Penn began in the early 1990s. Till then, almost all medical schools required two years of preclinical classroom work and two years of clinical work. But in 1989, Penn hired Bill Kelley away from the University of Michigan to serve as dean of the School of Medicine.

Bill had done his internship at the University of Texas Southwestern Medical Center, where his mentor was Donald Seldin. He was actually quite a conservative fellow, but the reforms he implemented at Penn altered medical education in a profoundly unconservative way.

When Bill arrived, Penn was ranked perhaps fifteenth in the nation: good, but not top tier. His goal was to put us into the top five in every category of medical education and research. And he damn near succeeded. By 1999, fourteen of the Perelman School of Medicine's "academic departments were ranked in the top 5 in their respective disciplines." And Penn's ranking in the annual *U.S. News & World Report* survey had rocketed up to third.[62]

Bill Kelley believed that medical students needed to cut back on the amount of time they spent in the classroom and instead spend more time getting out and taking care of patients. I thought it was a terrible idea, but I concede that running around and playing doctor is more "fun" than hitting the books. Bill thought this would make Penn more attractive to the top students, and perhaps he was right.

But the long-term consequences have been harmful. Nearly every medical school in the country has since adopted some variation on this model. Duke, for instance, a very fine school, offers just one year of classroom training, one year of research, and then a year and a half of clinical work, and that's it.

At Penn and many other schools now, the first four months of a medical student's course of study are devoted to basic science but merged with clinical science. They'll learn genetics, immunology, anatomy, neuroscience, and biochemistry initially. They then learn about disease and about normal function in integrated courses that are organ-based. For example, instead of a course in basic physiology that covers cellular function in the various organs in great detail, they now learn about the anatomy, cell function, and diseases of the heart in one six-week segment. This "saves time" and avoids learning more detailed aspects of the topic, but there is a real cost. The details are important and the deeper

---

[62] Edward W. Holmes, MD, "Of rice and men: Bill Kelley's next generation," *Journal of Clinical Investigation* 115, no. 10 (2005): 2948–2952.

the background information, the more students are able to incorporate newly developed knowledge into their later clinical practice. Often, what sounds like an obscure detail becomes the basis for a whole new approach to treatment in later years.

Thus, by the end of the first fourteen months they have gone through the major organ systems and had a smattering of basic science. Then it's off to clinical rotations, where lectures in surgery and other advanced subjects augment the clinical experience. The aspiring doctors are not given a textbook on surgery and told to read the damn thing, as we were in days long gone.

We used to buy textbooks, read them, and then buy auxiliary books to aid in understanding the textbooks. There's not even a bookstore at Penn's medical school anymore. Textbooks have become an anachronism on the order of handheld Texas Instruments calculators. And the library is now a lonely place. Lectures are recorded, and at the conclusion of the class the instructor gives a summary lecture on the material that will be on the exam.

At the majority of medical schools—including Penn, over my objections—numerical grades have given way to the pass/fail system in preclinical years. As a result, the attrition rate at Penn and across the nation's medical schools is now about 3 percent, as opposed to 9–10 percent in the bad old days.

Students still work hard, but realizing that all one has to do is scrape by with a "pass" means they are more conscious about achieving a work/life balance. This is no doubt a healthy goal for most people, but the life of a medical student is insanely busy, and that, we have found over decades of experience, is how it should be if we are to train the best possible physicians. Gone are the days when Dr. Donald Seldin told med students who had failed to do their homework, "Here's a dime. Call your mother. Only she can love you now."[63]

---

[63]   Schuster, "Donald W. Seldin, MD (1920–2018)," 439.

Getting into a highly recognized training program for your specialty remains a goal for many medical students. This was incredibly competitive. Penn, for instance, had fifteen or so slots in my internship group. The applicants for these highly selective positions numbered upwards of three hundred.

Before pass/fail, the only way you were earning one of these coveted posts was by working your way to the top of your class, grade-wise, and getting outstanding recommendations. These recommendations were not shared with students, which means they were usually very frank and even painfully honest. The interview with a panel of physicians could be grueling; they'd grill you with medical questions and you would answer to the best of your ability.

Today, grades have been demoted in importance, especially in pass/fail schools. Recommendations, even when putatively confidential, are always risky, for offering a less than hearty assessment of a student can cause headaches or unpleasantness down the road. With respect to the interview, the tables have turned. It has become akin to recruitment, as the panel tries to convince the student, especially if he or she belongs to a desired demographic category, to grace the school with his or her presence. The toughest question the applicant is likely to be asked is the cliché-grooved softball, "What challenges have you overcome in your life?"

Medical school is no longer any kind of barrier or winnowing funnel to a career as a doctor; it is more a pathway. Once on the path, it's hard to be derailed. In fact, accrediting agencies will sanction a school if too many students drop or flunk out. Rather than being a sign of a difficult, challenging environment, a high attrition rate is regarded as evidence that the school is insufficiently supportive of its students. It doesn't hold their hands or wipe their noses enough.

We expect some members of society to be totally devoted to their responsibilities and to sacrifice their own comfort for others. Think of Navy Seals, firefighters, airline pilots, and other first responders. We expect them to be wholly committed to their tasks and to those they serve. We should expect the same from physicians. Their education and training must prepare them for that sort of commitment. Unfortunately, that is no longer the case.

The accreditors also survey students to find out how happy they are and whether anyone has been nasty or disrespectful toward them. Heaven forbid that a tough, exacting teacher who demands excellence hurts someone's feelings! The whole thing is crazy: the goal has shifted from turning out the best physicians to turning out the happiest new physicians.

As mentioned, the attrition rate in US med schools has averaged just over 3 percent for the last quarter-century. In recent times, "more medical students left medical school due to nonacademic reasons than due to academic reasons," according to the AAMC.[64] Another study, this one of thirty-three thousand medical students, found that between 2014 and 2016 the percentage of black students who left med school (5.7 percent) was more than twice that of white students (2.3 percent).[65]

This is not to say that medical schools are not producing talented and dedicated doctors. Most graduates are just that. They work hard. But the reforms of the last generation mean that we are turning out more subpar doctors than ever before.

Two things, however, have helped. Residencies have improved, in part due to the deficiencies I have just mentioned. Physicians are so poorly trained in medical school that the educational component of residency programs has been beefed up in response. Lectures and academic expectations for the trainees have bolstered the quality of most residencies. But it is also true that the residency programs push much harder for "diversity," even in the face of surpassingly few opportunities for training. In ophthalmology and dermatology, there may be one hundred

[64] "Graduation Rates and Attrition Rates of U.S. Medical Students," Association of American Medical Colleges, AAMC Student Records System, October 2023.

[65] Jacqueline Howard, "Only 5.75% of US doctors are Black, and experts warn the shortage harms public health," CNN Health, February 21, 2023.

aspirants for every opening. If you're white or Asian, you'd better be a superstar.

The incredible advances in imaging and technology are the second boon to medical education. When I was in medical school, if someone came in complaining of abdominal pain, all you could do is listen and order an X-ray. The X-ray would not reveal anything about the internal workings of the abdomen. It would merely tell you if there was a kidney stone or similar mass. In the absence of such revelation, you had to call upon your training in how abdominal problems present in order to make a diagnosis.

Today, an MRI or CAT scan will show you exactly what's going on. They're not perfect, but they take us much further along the path. Someone who staggers into an emergency room moaning with right lower-quadrant pain isn't diagnosed with appendicitis because of her symptoms; instead, she gets diagnosed because the CAT scan shows an inflamed appendix. This, as well as advances in laboratory testing, has made an enormous difference for the better.

Some DEI proponents argue that the technological progress nullifies the critics' case because medical care is better than ever before. They're wrong. Consider the studies of autopsy accuracy. When I was a student, there was generally a 30–40 percent mismatch between autopsy results and clinical diagnosis. So in about a third of the cases which required an autopsy, the doctors had gotten it wrong. (It should be pointed out that autopsies have become relatively rare. Whereas in 1972, 19.1 percent of deaths were autopsied, that number fell to 9.4 percent in 1994 and has remained below 10 percent ever since.[66] Today, despite far superior technology, the misdiagnosis rate remains about the same as it was half a century or more ago. This suggests a decline in the diagnostic ability of the doctors our medical schools are turning out.)

---

[66] Donna L. Hoyert, "Autopsies in the United States in 2020," *National Vital Statistics Report* 72, no. 5 (May 24, 2023): 2.

- - - - - -

The website of the University of North Carolina School of Medicine tells applicants that "smart is easy."[67] This is flatly untrue, unless the student pool is drawn from Garrison Keillor's Lake Wobegon, where all the children are above average. But untruths are in the saddle these days.

Dr. Darrell Kirch, then-president of the AAMC, announced in 2011, "I am a man on a mission. I believe it is critical to our future to transform health care. I'm not talking about tweaking it. I'm not talking about some nuanced improvements here and there. I'm talking about true transformation."[68]

This sweeping transformation included revisions to the Medical College Admission Test (MCAT), the gold-standard exam that measures students' grasp of and aptitude for the life-saving profession.[69] It now "screens for progressive orthodoxies," noted Devorah Goldman of the Ethics and Public Policy Center. As illustration, one 2018 AAMC/Khan Academy MCAT practice question asked the reason for the "lack of minorities such as African Americans or Latinos/Latinas among university faculty members." The question did not permit open-ended answers. Rather, the test-taker had to choose between symbolic racism, institutional racism, hidden racism, or personal bias. Even the dimmest bulbs got the drift. The preferred AAMC answer, by the way, was institutional racism.[70]

Until recently, unless exceptional circumstances obtained, medical school applicants needed to exceed a certain grade point average and score on the MCAT to earn admittance. These floors are variable: whites

---

[67]   "Our Ideal Candidate," University of North Carolina School of Medicine, https://www.med.unc.edu/admit/requirements/our-ideal-candidate/, accessed September 1, 2022.

[68]   Letters, "The Political Transformation of Medicine," *Wall Street Journal*, April 24, 2022.

[69]   The first iteration of the MCAT appeared in 1928 in response to medical-school attrition rates as high as 50%. William C. McGaghie, "Assessing readiness for medical education: evolution of the medical college admission test," *Journal of the American Medical Association* 288, no. 9 (September 2002): 1085–1090.

[70]   Goldman, "The Politicization of the MCAT."

and Asians who post average scores are out of luck, but black and certain other minority med-school hopefuls have an excellent chance of admission even with middling GPA and MCAT scores.

Alarmingly, to fight alleged "systemic racism" at least forty institutions have dropped the MCAT requirement.[71] Even Penn's Perelman School of Medicine waives the MCAT for a number of applicants each year, primarily graduates of historically black colleges and universities (HBCUs). This keeps the school's average MCAT numbers high, but it puts these HBCU students in a tough place. They are given remedial instruction before school commences, but studies show that at many schools these students have higher dropout rates than their classmates.

Mark Perry, a senior fellow at Do No Harm and a professor of economics at the University of Michigan-Flint, has published data previously supplied by the AAMC showing that black applicants with average GPAs and average MCAT scores were almost four times more likely to be admitted to US medical schools than Asian applicants and three times more likely than white applicants with similar scores. Down the ladder the gap was even more glaring. Black applicants with lower-than-average GPAs and MCAT scores had a likelihood of admission that was nine times greater than comparable Asians and seven times greater than comparable white applicants. All white and Asian applicants with substandard performance had a 16.7 percent chance of acceptance, while blacks with a similar below-average performance had an 86 percent rate of acceptance.[72]

While I firmly believe—and have seen—that people of all backgrounds can become great physicians, I also believe that high standards are essential to identifying the most promising students. Medical schools

71   Akhil Katakam, "Medical Schools That Don't Require the MCAT: Top Programs List," Inspira Advantage, July 29, 2024, https://www.inspiraadvantage.com/blog/medical-schools-that-dont-require-the-mcat-what-you-should-know.

72   Mark Perry, "New Chart Illustrates Graphically the Racial Preferences for Blacks, Hispanics Being Admitted to US Medical Schools," American Enterprise Institute, June 25, 2017, https://www.aei.org/carpe-diem/new-chart-illustrates-graphically-racial-preferences-for-blacks-and-hispanics-being-admitted-to-us-medical-schools/.

should be strengthening those standards for everyone, not weakening them for any one group.

Denying opportunity to people on the basis of their skin color or genetic makeup is just plain wrong.

Elite schools that boast of a double-digit percentage of black medical students are being disingenuous. A disproportionate number of their black students hail from Africa or the Caribbean. True African Americans, especially African American males, are harder to find at such places.

A lot of the minority admittees are from the middle class or above. There is a case to be made for affirmative action based on poverty or social class; students from poor or disadvantaged backgrounds may well deserve a leg up, a special boost. But to see the children of affluent parents get into school simply because of the color of their skin is absolutely enraging. Schools boast of the number of students they admit from underrepresented-in-medicine categories, which leads to absurdities like Julio Rosenbaum (I have changed his name), a rich kid from Argentina, being counted as a URIM Hispanic medical student.

If a Chinese American kid and the white son of a grocery-store clerk who ace their MCATs are rejected, while a Nigerian diplomat's son, who has a lower score on his MCAT, is ushered in, it's not right. And until Do No Harm came on the scene, there was no organizational voice speaking up for justice in the medical space.

An applicant's DEI profile is becoming a factor in admissions decisions as well. When Do No Harm's Laura Morgan reviewed the admissions process at fifty of the top-ranked medical schools in the country, she found that thirty-six of them, or fully 72 percent, asked applicants about their views of or experience with DEI efforts. (These DEI questions are asked on what are known as secondary applications, which vary by school; applicants submit a primary application through the American Medical College Application Service.)

In some cases the ideological bias of these crucial secondary applications is so explicit as to rival political litmus tests in the old Soviet bloc nations.

Think I'm exaggerating?

Consider these questions asked of med-school applicants:

— "We are interested in combating all forms of systemic barriers, and would like to hear your thoughts on opposing specifically: systemic racism, anti-LGBTQ+ discrimination, and misogyny. How will you contribute?"—University of Pittsburgh School of Medicine

— "Do you identify as being part of a group that has been marginalized (examples include, but are not limited to, LGBTQIA, disabilities, federally recognized tribe) in terms of access to education or healthcare? If so, describe how this inequity has impacted you or your community and how educational disparity, health disparity and/or marginalization has impacted you and your community."—David Geffen School of Medicine at UCLA

— "The OSU COM Admissions vision statement states that the admissions committee will assemble a class that displays 'diversity in background and thought.' Why is 'diversity in background and thought' a desirable characteristic for a medical school's student body?"—The Ohio State University College of Medicine

— "Our country is reckoning with its history, racism, racial injustice, and especially anti-black racism. Please share your reflections on, experiences with, and greatest lessons learned about systemic racism."—University of Minnesota Medical School

— "What have you done to help identify, address and correct an issue of systemic discrimination?"—University of Miami Miller School of Medicine

This tendentiousness does not stop at the Top 50. Less prestigious medical schools are no less overt in their bias. For instance, Florida Atlantic University's Charles E. Schmidt College of Medicine hectors applicants, "As a future medical student at FAU, how can you play an active role in addressing and dismantling systemic racism?"

Those who have not imbibed deeply of the DEI Kool-Aid have limited options in answering such questions, and none of them are good. They can cynically tell the admissions committee what it wants to hear, thereby beginning their medical career with a lie. They can skirt the question, answering it only indirectly, thereby weakening their application. Or they can be true to themselves, challenging or disagreeing with the premise of the question, and thereby ensure that their application is quickly dispatched to the Rejection pile.

As Laura Morgan notes, the intent of including such questions is to make clear to applicants that support of DEI philosophy and initiatives is a credential that improves one's chances of acceptance to medical school. In this way dissenters are discouraged from applying, and those who make their dissent known are effectively screened out.

One winces to imagine the naïve applicant who, when asked about his or her personal experiences with diversity, begins a response with:

— "As a person from a small town..."
— "As a fundamentalist Christian..."
— "As an Orthodox Jew..."
— "As a Republican..."

Laura says, "Many questions cross a clear line from asking applicants to describe their background and life experiences to demanding their explicit support and enthusiasm for a worldview and agenda that is fundamentally political in nature. These demands for endorsement of specific political ideas in order to be considered for admission may constitute, or be close to constituting, compelled speech—a long-recognized violation of our country's most basic values of free speech and freedom of conscience."

She concludes: "Top medical schools have woven their commitment to woke politics into their application process, asking future doctors to prove their commitment to divisive ideologies or risk being rejected from medical school."[73]

We will never know how many lives might have been saved or extended by men and women who were blocked from becoming doctors by failing DEI litmus tests.

Follow the evidence is a foundational tenet of healthcare, as it is of all scientific inquiry. Yet today's medical establishment is unwilling to confront the consequences of its attempts to maximize diversity. After years of lowering standards for applicants, medical schools are more diverse than ever before. In the 2023–24 academic year, one in ten medical school applicants was black or African American. Over 55 percent were female, meaning men are now an "underrepresented in medicine" group.[74]

Yet several new studies show that many minority students are struggling, putting their future patients and careers at risk. Rather than revisit the means by which they are pursuing diversity, however, the medical elite want to double down on their failing course.

The campaign for diversity has some value, but the ideological extremism of the DEI craze has led medical schools to adopt dangerous strategies, ranging from scrapping letter grades in favor of the lax "pass/fail" binary to dropping the requirement that applicants take the MCAT.

It's also getting harder to gauge whether graduates are well prepared. The US Medical Licensing Exam, which residencies rely on when picking trainees, recently abandoned objective grading for a pass/fail system,

[73]   Laura L. Morgan, "Only DEI Advocates Need Apply," Do No Harm, August 2022.
[74]   Association of American Medical Colleges, "New AAMC Data on Diversity in Medical School Enrollment in 2023," press release, December 12, 2023.

largely on diversity grounds. And calls are growing for post-graduate resident evaluations to be weakened as well. That would let potentially unqualified individuals enter medical practice and endanger patient well-being.

As I said in the introduction, further research has confirmed the validity of the question I tweeted to such an outrageous response in 2022. A study published in *Academic Medicine* demonstrated that those who perform better on exams perform better as physicians. This may seem like a commonplace observation, a dog-bites-man story, but it goes against the grain. It is contentious not because of the evidence, which readily affirms its truth, but because of the implications.

The researchers parsed data from US and Canadian MD-granting medical schools to examine the predictive validity of MCAT scores and undergraduate grade point averages for medical student performance at several junctures of a doctor's education. Specifically, these were pre-clerkship and clerkship courses, the first two (of three) steps in the US Medical Licensing Examination, and in medical school.

Not surprisingly, the researchers found that MCAT scores generally predict student outcomes. Those with lower scores fare worse over their four years in the classroom, and the strong correlation between MCAT scores and student success holds across racial, ethnic, and socioeconomic lines.

The authors inserted the non sequitur sentence "The importance of diversifying the physician workforce is undeniable," perhaps as a talisman against potential charges of wrongthink.[75] You can't be too careful these days.

Additionally, a 2023 study of 634 assessments made of 2,708 emergency medicine residents in 128 ACGME-accredited programs found that while there were "no statistically significant differences in

---

[75] Joshua Hanson et al., "The Validity of MCAT Scores in Predicting Students' Performance and Progress in Medical School: Results From a Multisite Study," *Academic Medicine* 97, no. 9 (September 2022): 1374–1384.

assessments between White male and female residents," URIM female residents were rated significantly lower in all six competencies: patient care, medical knowledge, systems-based practice, practice-based learning and improvement, professionalism, and interpersonal and communication skills.

The authors give one and only one possible reason for the disparity: "intersectional discrimination in physician competency evaluation." The complete and utter lack of curiosity about other possible explanations gives off the timorous vibe of writers deathly afraid of violating some orthodoxy, punishment for which is professional death.[76]

And a relevant study was published by the news site STAT just days after my infamous tweet. In a thorough investigation of post-graduate residencies, it found that black residents "either leave or are terminated from training programs at far higher rates than white residents."

The author concluded that the "result of this culling—long hidden, dismissed, and ignored by the larger medical establishment—is that many Black physicians have been unable to enter lucrative and extremely white specialties such as neurosurgery, dermatology, or plastic surgery."

STAT assumed that racism accounts for this disparity, but the other studies point to a simpler and more credible explanation: after struggling in medical school and falling short in key professional indicators, some residents simply lose their positions due to poor performance. As a longtime medical educator, I can attest that no training program would make this difficult and disruptive decision for any reason other than competence and concern for patients.[77]

Such findings should spark a diversity rethink among medical school administrators. They should be deeply concerned that they're accepting and graduating a growing number of students who may not be ready for

---

[76] Elle Lett et al., "Intersectional Disparities in Emergency Medicine Residents' Performance Assessments by Race, Ethnicity, and Sex," *JAMA Network Open* 6, no. 9 (2023).

[77] Usha Lee McFarling, "'It was stolen from me': Black doctors are forced out of training programs at far higher rates than white residents," STAT, June 20, 2022.

the rigors of the profession. They should also be concerned that more qualified students are likely being passed over, leaving patients with a less talented crop of doctors over the long run.

But a rethink is not what medical schools want. That would require questioning the ideological assumption that patients need to see physicians of the same race and gender, an idea contradicted by robust clinical studies. More to the point, it would call into question the entire diversity-industrial complex. This ideology runs so deep that I doubt medical schools will put student quality ahead of diversity unless policymakers require it, either by mandating the MCAT for all students or withholding funding from institutions that put skin color ahead of medical excellence.

People of every race and background are fully capable of becoming world-class physicians. Medical schools should seek out the best candidates who are most likely to provide the best care for patients, regardless of what they look like or where they come from. Anything less jeopardizes the very purpose of these institutions. The medical elite may not want to admit it, but their current approach to achieving diversity has a steep cost, and it's wrong to ask patients to pay it.

The evidence is irrefutable: grades and assessments are not irrelevant. A 2024 study of 6,898 hospitalists published in the *Journal of the American Medical Association* found that higher scores on the certification exam administered by the American Board of Internal Medicine was associated with "reduced 7-day mortality and readmissions."[78] In other words, the lower a doctor's scores on the certifying exam, the greater the likelihood that his or her patients will die. That's pretty stark.

Numerous studies suggest a strong predictive value in the MCAT. Performance in medical school predicts how well you do as a resident, and performance as a resident predicts how well you do as a practicing

---

[78] Bradley M. Gray et al., "Associations of Internal Medicine Residency Milestone Ratings and Certification Examination Scores with Patient Outcomes," *JAMA* 332, no. 4 (2024): 300–309.

physician. Eliminating MCAT requirements, basing admission on inflated undergraduate grades, and deciding that holistic admissions rather than rigorous assessment of academic potential is the way to determine who should have the opportunity to be a physician will inevitably lead to less effective healthcare.

Everyone knows this, but no one wants to talk about it. Avoiding a hassle is a great motivator of inaction and silence.

If you go to Harvard hospitals and ask around, you'll find that the physicians are pleased with the quality of the newly minted minority doctors. But they are getting the best of the best. Go to a state school whose medical school is only five or ten years old and you'll get a different story. They'll have some very weak students who will become doctors—hardly anyone flunks out anymore—but very weak doctors. You sure as hell don't want them on duty when you're taken to the emergency room in the middle of the night.

CHAPTER FOUR

THE WOKEST OF THE WOKE: NAMING NAMES

In November 2022, the Association of American Medical Colleges released *The Power of Collective Action: Assessing and Advancing Diversity, Equity, and Inclusion Efforts at AAMC Medical Schools*, its first-ever analysis of the extent to which DEI has infected the institutions training future physicians. It was even worse than I'd expected.

The AAMC surveyed 101 institutions, representing almost two-thirds of American medical schools (two of those surveyed were Canadian), asking for audits of their DEI-related policies and programs: what they called the Diversity, Inclusion, Culture, and Equity (DICE) inventory. (DICE does have a better ring to it than DEI, which mischievous souls transpose to DIE.)

Do No Harm discovered the existence of the DICE audit when The Ohio State University included the document prepared by its College of Medicine in response to our Freedom of Information Act request.

The AAMC asked medical schools to answer eighty-nine yes-or-no questions on whether they have specific DEI activities. The results are shown as a kind of report card. Schools that score 80 percent are colored green, and those that score between 61 percent and 80 percent are yellow. Institutions below the 60 percent threshold are red—the stop sign of failure.

Unfortunately for the patients of America, most medical schools aced the test. More than six in ten scored 80 percent. The Ohio State University College of Medicine audit shows a score of 93 percent, making it one of the most woke medical schools in America. (More on that soon.) Crucially, no institution scored lower than 50 percent—meaning virtually every medical school is implementing at least half the policies woke activists want.

In what areas are they wokest? Every single medical school in the survey practices affirmative action, which the AAMC redefines as "admissions policies and practices for encouraging a diverse class of students" instead of the more honest "discrimination against Asian and white applicants." Fully 85 percent have leaders who've "used demographic data to promote change" within their institution. What this vague formulation means is that medical schools are giving skin color and gender a consistently bigger emphasis in recruiting. This approach risks deprioritizing merit, leading to a lower quality of medical students and worse care for the 100 percent of Americans who at some point take ill.

Schools are all but uniformly woke on many other measures. Ninety-nine percent have leaders who routinely participate in local, state, or national DEI forums, diverting their focus from actual education. Some 98 percent have created a system for students to report bias—that is, act as tattletales and snitches—which risks self-censorship from educators who fear reprisal for teaching healthcare's more difficult topics. The same percentage have launched new initiatives or funding streams for DEI, while 97 percent have "a dedicated office, staff, and resources" for this ulcerous ideology.

That means there's a permanent bureaucracy at most medical schools pushing woke ideology on faculty and students alike. These efforts take away time and money from actual education.

Where are medical schools falling short on the woke checklist? "Only" 75 percent advocate for DEI "policies and/or legislation at a local, state, or federal level." Yet that means three out of four medical schools are using precious resources (and their powerful clout) to push a divisive politicized agenda. A good example is The Ohio State University's support for declaring racism a public-health crisis in its home city of Columbus. This also wastes resources that would be better spent on medical training.

More than 40 percent of medical schools—including the Indiana University School of Medicine, which we'll meet later this chapter—offer tenure and promotions to faculty who conduct DEI scholarship. The message to current and potential faculty is clear: if you want to advance in your career, you'd better toe the party line. Yet more biased papers on DEI mean fewer on pressing issues in cardiology, nephrology, dermatology, and other less sexy but infinitely more important subjects.

The AAMC is not a lax class monitor when it comes to DEI. It is pushing 100 percent of medical schools to score 100 percent in each category—and most are trending in that direction. This doesn't bode well for the future of healthcare. Medical schools are broadly lowering standards for admissions, faculty, and research while devoting a higher share of resources to political lobbying, politicized bureaucracy, and public virtue signaling.

Is there any way to stop this trend?

Yes. For starters, governors or legislatures should require every medical school in their state that participated in the AAMC report to publish its audit. Then lawmakers should hold hearings on the findings. Ultimately, they should evaluate whether these medical schools deserve so much state money.

Why are taxpayers funding schools that only recruit politicized faculty? Why are they paying administrators who fixate on applicants' skin color? The public deserves to know exactly how woke their nearest medical school is so they can pressure it to put education—and ultimately the quality of care—ahead of ideology.[79]

Perhaps no once-respected medical school has sunk so deeply into DEI madness as UCLA's David Geffen School of Medicine.

Washington Free Beacon investigative reporter Aaron Sibarium produced an eye-opening, jaw-dropping account of how the Geffen School's dean of admissions, Jennifer Lucero, has presided over UCLA's precipitous fall. As one former admissions staffer told Sibarium, UCLA has become a "failed medical school" because "we want racial diversity so badly, we're willing to cut corners to get it."

Although in 1996 California voters outlawed affirmative action based on race, sex, or ethnicity by approving Proposition 209, the California Civil Rights Initiative, UCLA has thumbed its institutional nose at the will of the voters. Faculty members, admissions staff, and others with direct knowledge of UCLA policy told Sibarium that in recent years the med school has admitted grossly unqualified students. "All the normal criteria for getting into medical school only apply to people of certain races," said an admissions officer. "For other people, those criteria are completely disregarded."

The number of UCLA med students who fail shelf exams, which assess student knowledge at the end of clinical clerkships in such areas as family medicine, pediatrics, and internal medicine, has increased as much as tenfold in some subjects since Lucero took over as admissions dean in 2020. In 2021, one-quarter of UCLA med students flunked at least three shelf exams.

One frustrated UCLA med school professor told Sibarium, "I don't know how some of these students are going to be junior doctors. Faculty

---

79   Stanley Goldfarb, "Med schools are even more woke than you think—and your care is at risk," *New York Post*, November 16, 2022.

are seeing a shocking decline in knowledge of medical students." Exacerbating the damage done by a DEI-obsessed admissions dean is the fact that UCLA reduced its "preclinical curriculum from two years to one in order to add more time for research and community service."

Four members of the admissions committee told Sibarium that it "routinely gives black and Latino applicants a pass for subpar metrics," while "whites and Asians need near perfect scores to even be considered." One of those committee members said that the bar for underrepresented-in-medicine minorities to be admitted to UCLA is "as low as you could possibly imagine."

When an admissions officer questioned whether "a black applicant with grades and test scores far below the UCLA average" should be admitted, Lucero went ballistic. "Did you not know African-American women are dying at a higher rate than everybody else?" she shouted. Just how the admission of an unqualified student will extend the life of even one African American woman went unexplained.

Numerous complaints have been lodged against Lucero, but the UCLA Discrimination Prevention Office apparently thinks discrimination only runs one way. One complaint cited Lucero for demanding "that a highly qualified white male be knocked down several spots because, as she put it, 'we have too many of his kind' already." She also dismissed objections from doctors because they were "not BIPOC (Black, Indigenous, and People of Color)." Sounds like a charming woman.

The *Free Beacon* article is devastating—and depressing. We are witnessing the destruction of a once-proud medical school. As one med school professor told Aaron Sibarium, "UCLA still produces some very good graduates, but a third to a half of the medical school is incredibly unqualified."[80]

---

[80] Aaron Sibarium, "'A Failed Medical School': How Racial Preferences, Supposedly Outlawed in California, Have Persisted at UCLA," *Washington Free Beacon*, May 23, 2024.

- - - - - -

An increasing number of med schools are refusing to share data with *U.S. News & World Report*, claiming that "the magazine's annual rankings hinder their ability to increase diversity." One such, New York's Icahn School of Medicine at Mount Sinai, explains that these rankings punish schools for their "commitment to anti-racism, and outreach to diverse communities."

Writing in the *Wall Street Journal*, Fritz François and Gbenga Ogedegbe of New York University's Grossman School of Medicine opine, "What these schools are really saying is that meritocracy can't coexist with diversity. This is a presumptuous—and dangerous—perpetuation of the negative stereotype that students from backgrounds that are underrepresented in medicine are of lesser quality or unable to compete."[81]

It is also an admission that schools struggle to maintain excellence while pursuing politicized demands for racial diversity in their student bodies.

There is no evidence that minority students who are qualified to enter medical school are being denied admission. While the Liaison Committee on Medical Education has required medical schools to increase the diversity of their classes for several years, the number of minority students has increased only minimally and remains well below the sought-after goal of equaling the proportion of blacks in America. Medical schools have had to confront the fact that an insufficient number of qualified students are available. Forcing greater diversity therefore must lead to a reduction in the merit of the students accepted.

Pursuing this approach will only undermine the academic achievements of those minority students who deserve admission to medical school and want eagerly to pursue a career in medicine. They deserve fair treatment, just as patients deserve the highest standard of care.

---

[81] Fritz François and Gbenga Ogedegbe, "Medical Schools Are Wrong to Think Diversity and Merit Are in Conflict," *Wall Street Journal*, February 15, 2023.

It is difficult to have good-faith discussions about such matters with the hierarchs of med schools, as they speak and write in such spiritless jargon that it may as well have been composed by an AI program. They speak of "dismantling structures and systems that perpetuate inequalities that lead to differential health outcomes…for black, Latinx, and indigenous populations" without bothering to prove such a linkage. (The use of *Latinx* is a failsafe tipoff. The term is detested by most Spanish-speaking people, who resent the attempt by imperious mandarins of the professional academic class to impose it upon them.)[82]

Dr. David J. Skorton, president and CEO of the Association of American Medical Colleges, and Dr. Henri R. Ford, dean of the University of Miami medical school and chairman of the AAMC's council of deans, responded to an op-ed of mine in the *Wall Street Journal* using this kind of woke boilerplate:

> Our goal, and that of every medical school, is to recruit a diverse class of talented medical students in a holistic fashion and educate them to improve the health of their patients and communities. There is ample evidence that historically marginalized people who live in poverty, as well as members of LGBTQ communities, disproportionately experience poor health and inadequate access to quality care. These inequities are often rooted in systemic discrimination, including racism.[83]

While the disparities are real, their explanation for them is fantasy.

---

[82] Letters, "How a Hospital Thinks About Systemic Racism," *Wall Street Journal*, May 2, 2022.

[83] Letters, "Why We Educate for Equity at Medical School," *Wall Street Journal*, April 28, 2022; Stanley Goldfarb, "Keep Politics Out of the Doctor's Office," *Wall Street Journal*, April 18, 2022.

I went through two accreditation cycles at Penn. Even at the first, which was in 2008, the Liaison Committee on Medical Education, the accrediting body, required us to meet a diversity standard and explain what steps we had taken to meet it. (The LCME is a joint project of the AMA and the AAMC.)

The accreditation process is big on bark but weak on bite. It's fake in many ways. Everyone knows that the LCME is not going to take away Perelman's accreditation if the percentage of black or Pacific Islander or Latino students fails to reach an arbitrary threshold. But woke bureaucrats within the school use that specious threat to get their way. They warn that dire consequences await if the school does not bend to their will, and no one ever calls their bluff.

For example, the Liaison Committee on Medical Education stipulates that medical schools must engage in "ongoing, systematic, and focused recruitment and retention activities, to achieve mission-appropriate diversity outcomes." This sounds harsh and forbidding. Members of Congress wanted to know more.

So on May 4, 2023, Representative Virginia Foxx (R-NC), chairwoman of the US House Committee on Education and the Workforce; Representative Burgess Owens (R-UT), chairman of the committee's Subcommittee on Higher Education and Workforce Development; and two of their colleagues sent a letter to Dr. Barbara Barzansky, the AMA's cosecretary of the LCME; and Dr. Veronica M. Catanese, the AAMC's cosecretary of the LCME. They questioned the Liaison Committee on Medical Education's "commitment to ensuring that medical schools are preparing future health care professionals to provide healthcare free from racial discrimination."

It was a classic case of calling a bully's bluff—and winning.

The congressional quartet noted that Standard 3 of the LCME's accreditation standards required that medical schools "recogniz[e] the benefits of diversity," and Element 3.3 of Standard 3 demanded "mission-appropriate diversity outcomes" that may be achieved by "the use of programs and/or partnerships aimed at achieving diversity among qualified applicants."

What did this mass of verbiage mean? Specifically, asked Reps. Foxx, Owens, et al.:

1. Does LCME require and/or encourage medical schools to treat applicants differently based on the applicants' race?
2. Does LCME require and/or encourage medical schools to award scholarships based on recipients' race?
3. Can a medical school satisfy Element 3.3 if the school chooses to treat its applicants, students, faculty, and staff equally, irrespective of their race?
4. Can a medical school satisfy Standard 3 if the school chooses to treat its applicants, students, faculty, and staff equally, irrespective of their race?
5. Does LCME require and/or encourage medical schools to teach that it is preferable for doctors and patients to be the same race?
6. In LCME's view, is it preferable for doctors and patients to be the same race?
7. Does LCME require or encourage medical schools to teach that the American health care system is systemically racist?
8. In LCME's view, is the American health care system systemically racist?
9. Please describe all communications regarding racial diversity that LCME has published or sent in the past three years.
10. In LCME's view, are members of a particular race inherently racist or privileged?
11. In LCME's view, are members of a particular race inherently oppressed?

12. What steps does LCME take to pursue racial diversity in its own operations?
13. Does LCME pursue any antiracism efforts?
14. What percentage of LCME's budget is spent on diversity, equity, and inclusion initiatives?[84]

The cosecretaries' response was blandly conciliatory and seemed to give the LCME's blessing to race-blind reforms. They responded that "diversity" is open to interpretation and should not be construed as a statement about race.[85] They ran from DEI dogma like a kid fleeing from a window he had just broken.

The LCME letter put the kibosh on the idea that purging divisive and discriminatory woke ideology from medical schools would jeopardize a school's accreditation. That threat was a paper tiger.

When you stand up to bullies, sometimes they back down.

As the *Wall Street Journal* explained:

> LCME is now [signaling] its diversity requirement is not as inflexible as schools have assumed. In a letter responding to a questionnaire from the House Committee on Education and the Workforce, LCME says that "nothing" in the text "mandates which categories of diversity a medical school must use to satisfy this element." That's an opening for Missouri, Tennessee, Utah and other states looking for ways to get the DEI bureaucracy out of medical schools.[86]

[84] Virginia Foxx et al., Letter to LCME on Nondiscrimination, Committee on Education and the Workforce, May 4, 2023, https://edworkforce.house.gov/uploadedfiles/5.4.23_letter_to_lcme_on_nondiscrimination.pdf.
[85] Barbara Barzansky and Veronica M. Catanese, LCME Response, May 8, 2023, https://donoharmmedicine.org/wp-content/uploads/2023/07/Ltr-LCME-Response-May-18-2023.pdf.
[86] Editorial Board, "A Medical School Treatment for DEI," *Wall Street Journal*, July 25, 2023.

The LCME also disavowed pursuing so-called "anti-racism efforts," which, despite the name, require racial discrimination. The LCME denied that America is systemically racist and said it doesn't require medical schools to teach such a lie.

The message to state lawmakers couldn't have been clearer: there's nothing blocking them from getting woke ideology out of medical schools. Now that this threat is off the table, every state should pass sweeping reforms as soon as possible. Medical students—and the patients they will eventually treat—deserve swift action.[87]

The relatively laissez-faire attitude reflected in the LCME letter is not the way the committee's agents act when they visit your school. Those unwelcome encounters are more like getting a knock on the door from an IRS or FBI agent. You're not glad to see them, and they're not brimming with bonhomie and goodwill. If you don't have what they judge to be a sufficient number of faculty of color or a robust DEI program you will be chastised and threatened with a vaguely defined punishment.

If you do what they say, they'll leave you alone for eight years. If you are at all noncompliant, however, you'll have to go through the whole miserable routine again at a shorter interval, and it's a huge pain in the ass. It's nerve-wracking, harrowing, and expensive, as you have to hire high-priced consultants to guide you through the process. It's easier to just bow down and submit to the LCME's demands—but as the LCME itself has now admitted, you don't have to impose woke discrimination on your students and faculty.

---

[87] In 2024, Utah enacted the Equal Opportunities Initiative, which reined in DEI in a fashion that even the relatively liberal journal *The Atlantic* approved as a "promising" attempt to "end the excessive and at times coercive focus on identity in higher education while also trying to protect academic freedom with carve-outs for research and course teaching." Conor Friedersdorf, "The State That's Trying to Rein in DEI Without Becoming Florida," *The Atlantic*, March 31, 2024.

Junking the DEI infrastructure would do wonders for the quality and even social environment of US medical schools. As with communism or fascism, you won't eliminate the idea, but you will dramatically reduce the mischief and outright evil these bureaucracies do.

This goal is no pipe dream. Do No Harm's crack team of attorneys has crafted legislation to do just this, and our lobbyists are working receptive state legislatures to reduce or eliminate the malign influence of DEI offices in medical schools. Already, laws to scale back or even eliminate DEI in medical schools have been enacted in more than a dozen states.

There are states—California and New York, for instance—where legislatures are loath to reverse deleterious policies, but in those places our legal team explores ways to achieve justice by appealing to the state or federal constitutions.

You might think abolishing DEI would be a slam dunk, but the schools employ pricey lobbyists who keep the less diligent legislators happy with football tickets and other baubles. They are also not above dissembling, dissimulating, and outright lying to protect the sacred DEI cow. For instance, a Do No Harm–supported bill freeing the University of Tennessee of its DEI fiefdom was about to be approved by the relevant legislative committee when UT elicited a letter from the Knoxville Jewish Alliance arguing, nonsensically, that getting rid of DEI would harm Jewish students. The committee received this missive—whose assertion was the exact opposite of the truth—at the last minute, delaying passage for who knows how long.

This is just politics, they say: as ugly as sausage-making. But unfortunately, lives hang in the balance.

Do No Harm representatives, myself included, have testified on DEI legislation before state legislatures in Missouri, Kansas, Ohio, Utah, Arizona, Tennessee, and Texas. Typically, university lobbyists (whose munificent salaries are paid, of course, by the taxpayers) will feed compliant legislators hostile questions to ask us. They came after me for being "canceled" at the University of Pennsylvania, but the circumstances—I was canceled for criticizing egregious acts of DEI—are such that these attacks actually boost my image with most legislators.

There is a myth, propagated by the DEI industry, that federal civil rights laws require colleges and universities to operate DEI programs. False. Title VI and Title IX simply prohibit discrimination in education. Schools are not discriminating if they lack DEI programming, and DEI programming can even conflict with these laws by treating people differently based on race.

Texas and Florida have already enacted DEI bans in publicly funded institutions of higher education. The Texas law clarifies that publicly funded institutions of higher education "may not establish or maintain a diversity, equity, and inclusion office or hire or assign an employee of the institution, or contract with a third party, to perform the duties of a diversity, equity, and inclusion office." Similarly, Florida law now states that public universities "may not expend any state or federal funds to promote, support, or maintain any programs or campus activities that... advocate for diversity, equity, and inclusion, or promote or engage in political or social activism." Legislators in other states are mulling legislation along the same lines, and Do No Harm is in the forefront of this fight.

In addition to Texas and Florida, several states whose flagship medical schools are—or were—furthest gone in DEI lunacy are located in what the psephologists call "red states": North Carolina, Tennessee, Ohio, and Indiana.

Of the last-named, Indiana University School of Medicine graduate Dr. Cindy Basinski, a practicing physician and medical educator in the Hoosier State, told Do No Harm:

Every day, I talk with medical students and faculty at the IU School of Medicine. Their backgrounds and beliefs differ, but they all share the same concern. They see firsthand that IUSM is undermining medical education with divisive ideology. It's creating a culture of fear and self-censorship that harms them and, ultimately, patients across Indiana and beyond.

IUSM is going the same route as most medical schools nationwide, though it's arguably much further along the road.... Start with medical students. Before even getting into medical school, they are asked how they have promoted—or plan to promote—DEIJ [the J is for Justice] objectives. Students have also told me about the politicized lessons they get in the classroom. IUSM is downplaying medical science and ethics in favor of politicized narratives about race and gender.

Students don't dare disagree because they know it would destroy their chances of getting into residency programs they desire. They are completely dependent on recommendations from IUSM faculty, so they silence themselves for their own protection.

Faculty are also suffering. They cannot question the tenets of the DEIJ agenda, lest they be punished by administrators. Even worse, IUSM faculty are now required to show how they've advanced DEIJ in order to secure tenure or promotion. Whereas students are being forced into silence, IUSM faculty are being forced to be complicit with the corruption of medical education.

This runs counter to the purpose of medical education, the principles of medical science, and the pursuit of medical progress. The most incredible advances in medical history happened because students and faculty pushed the bounds of knowledge and questioned received wisdom. If faculty and future physicians aren't exposed to a wide variety of views, or even free to share their own perspectives, they won't move medicine forward. Patients will suffer.[88]

When cowed silence is the best option, you know that you're on the wrong path.

Among the unique projects undertaken by Do No Harm is a series of in-depth looks at the overt and insidious ways that woke politics and DEI have infected medical schools. Readers are welcome to access these reports, in all their gory and unconstitutional detail, on our website. I am pleased to say that state legislators and pro-freedom activists are making excellent use of this resource. Highlights (or, more properly, lowlights) from our series include:

The University of North Carolina at Chapel Hill School of Medicine's curriculum and educational experience are riddled and wracked with wokeism. The embrace of radical political ideologies by North Carolina's flagship medical school and the aggressiveness with which the school imposes them on students raise serious concerns for patients in North Carolina. They also generate questions about the rights of UNC-SOM medical students to pursue their education free from being compelled to participate in and express support for political causes.

The school's DEI office is Orwellian and intolerant, as such offices typically are. Its website greets viewers with a Black Lives Matter logo and shows young people wearing UNCSOM apparel and holding signs asserting, apodictically, such questionable claims as "Racism [is] a major

---

[88] "Indiana Doctor and Educator: IUSM Needs Immediate Reform," Do No Harm, September 5, 2023.

9 5

driver of health disparities," "Silence perpetuates violence," and "Speaking up is not enough: Allyship requires action."[89]

Students and faculty, be forewarned: dissent from these woke platitudes at your peril!

UNCSOM's Office of Diversity, Equity, and Inclusion is determined to "integrate social justice into the curriculum" and requires each department to develop an "Inclusive Excellence Plan." There are councils and committees, mandates and guidelines, and they go beyond empty gestures and rote recitals. For instance, UNCSOM's Departments of Biochemistry and Biophysics, Pharmacology, Nutrition, and Microbiology and Immunology have pledged themselves "committed to making meaningful changes in [our] operations to reduce demographic imbalances in the faculty and to contribute to dismantling the pervasive systemic racism that plagues academic research."[90]

What the reduction of demographic imbalances means is that the departments will discriminate against Asians and whites.

Do the taxpayers of North Carolina really want this?

The UNC medical school is big on panels and workshops about racial microaggressions. Lack of intent to microaggress is never a defense; the microaggressor is told he must apologize—even if he has no idea what the hell he is apologizing for.

The school also boasts that it is "a regional leader in transgender care," offering a "full range of urologic services including primary gender affirming surgery (including metoidioplasty, phalloplasty, and vaginoplasty), penile prosthesis, and orchiectomy." With a goal of "improv[ing] access to UNC Healthcare for transgender patients in the region," the

---

89 "The Path Forward," University of North Carolina School of Medicine, Office of Diversity, Equity, and Inclusion, https://www.med.unc.edu/inclusion/path-forward/, accessed September 1, 2022.

90 Documents released by UNCSOM in response to a Freedom of Information Act request by Do No Harm.

Department of Urology began the UNC Transgender Health Program.[91] UNCSOM does not limit transgender services to adults: its Pediatric and Adolescent Clinic for Gender Wellness has focused on providing "care to children and adolescents with gender dysphoria and other concerns."

In keeping with the general tone of Stalinist enforcement of woke ideology, faculty and students at UNCSOM are told to use inclusive language by "practic[ing] and us[ing] correct pronouns" and "tak[ing] correction with grace and humility." Lest there be any confusion, everyone at UNCSOM is instructed to "not express, reinforce or police 'the norm.'"[92]

Amidst the avalanche of material produced by UNC's School of Medicine extolling diversity and threatening punishment for those who don't toe the party line, one searches in vain for any mention of diversity of thought, religion, age, experience, or geography.

Do No Harm supporter Dr. Nancy Andersen, a graduate of Duke University and the George Washington University School of Medicine, did her general surgical residency at UNC School of Medicine. It was rigorous—and rigorously nonpolitical. As Nancy says:

> When I was in medical school and residency, we didn't talk about each other's politics. We tried to be objective and were focused on learning the best methods of care for our patients, not who our colleagues voted for.

That's why she was disheartened by the hard woke turn UNC's med school took. Her alumni newsletters featured stories about surgeons kneeling in social-justice protests, holding up Black Lives Matter signs, and supporting "gender affirming care."

---

91   "Urology Services for Transgender and Gender Diverse Individuals," University of North Carolina School of Medicine, Department of Urology, https://www.med.unc.edu/urology/transgender-health/, accessed September 1, 2022.

92   "Education," University of North Carolina School of Medicine, Health Sciences, https://www.med.unc.edu/healthsciences/ about-us/diversity/jeditoolkit/education/, accessed September 1, 2022.

Dr. Andersen's grandfather left Soviet-bloc Eastern Europe for the freedom of the United States. The stories he told his granddaughter about the evils of communism never left her. She understands the imperative of resistance.

When Dr. Andersen noticed the UNC pediatrics website promoted the 1619 Project curriculum and the "Genderbread Person" (a tool for trans proselytization among the young that is shaped like a gingerbread cookie) as resources for pediatrics, she alerted the media. UNC removed the references after significant backlash—proof that the bright light of publicity can have a cleansing effect. As can principled, effective legislation.[93]

The Ohio State University College of Medicine infuses healthy equity and "social justice" so thoroughly into its strategic plans that it seems bent on creating only health professionals who are agents of social change.

Its self-labeled "bold new curriculum" asserts that Ohio State medical students are part of the health-inequity problem due to their unexamined beliefs.

The bold new curriculum is necessary, according to Dean Carol R. Bradford, because the "lack of awareness and denial of racism within the profession of medicine relate in part to physicians not recognizing their negatively biased attitudes, perspectives and habits." First-years at OSUCOM are required to examine "the historical basis for some of the racist practices in medicine." Participants in this mandatory exercise take a pre-lecture survey to evaluate their "knowledge and attitudes about racism and racist beliefs," and then attend a lecture on the sources of "medical myths about African Americans that have been passed on as medical truths."[94]

---

[93] "Dr. Nancy Andersen," Do No Harm, https://donoharmmedicine.org/story/dr-nancy-andersen.

[94] "Anti-racism curriculum and assault victim curriculum," The Ohio State University College of Medicine, https://medicine.osu.edu/ why-choose-us/annual-report/antiracism-curriculum-and-assault-victim-curriculum, accessed June 12, 2023.

Ohio State takes thought control to the next level. The College of Medicine's Office of Diversity & Inclusion's *Resources for Taking Action Against Racism* hectors students on such subjects as "5 Do's and Don't's for White Leaders and Colleagues Discussing Racism at Work," "6 Questions to Stop Asking Your Black Friends and Colleagues Right Now," and "White Privilege in Health Care: Following Recognition with Action."[95]

Among the six questions that non-black students are told not to ask black colleagues is "How are you doing?"

Yes, that's right: The Ohio State University College of Medicine tells its staff, faculty, and students not to ask black colleagues and friends, "How are you doing?" The reason? "Black People (and all People of Color)...experience racism every day."[96]

Thankfully, not every state-supported school of medicine is as far gone as those in Ohio and North Carolina.

The pushback against DEI and what Elon Musk calls the "woke mind virus" is having an effect elsewhere. Take Florida, which is among the states whose legislature and governor are trying to root out DEI and its associated ideologies from public higher education, including medical school. This effort is still in the relatively early stages, but the legislation has been passed and signed, and the hard work of restoring political neutrality is underway.

State legislatures fund their public-university medical schools, which means they can also defund them. It is exceedingly unlikely—and undesirable—that a legislature will ever entirely defund a medical school, barring some catastrophic event, but state lawmakers can refuse to fund obnoxious programs, racially discriminatory policies, and the enforcement of such petty edicts as DEI pledges, which are a form of compelled

95   "Diversity and Inclusion: Resources for taking action against racism," The Ohio State University College of Medicine, https://medicine.osu.edu/diversity, accessed June 12, 2023.

96   Dynasti Hunt Harris, "6 questions to stop asking your black friends right now," *Medium*, May 31, 2020.

speech under which faculty members are forced to swear oaths to uphold the tenets of the diversity, equity, and inclusion sect.

Before the recent reforms in the Sunshine State, the University of Florida College of Medicine (UFCOM) notoriously infused DEI into seemingly all aspects of medical education. The conditioning began the moment a prospective student started exploring UFCOM, continued through the admissions process, and persisted throughout the doctoral program.

Do No Harm's 2022 report on UFCOM and DEI, written by Laura Morgan, found a medical school steeped in indoctrination. The Medical Admissions office at UFCOM made its first impression on visitors to its website by displaying a photograph of medical students on its main admissions landing page. This was not the usual stock image of carefully selected models simulating a conversation about a patient's diagnosis. Instead, the students' fists were raised high in the air, and they held a sign that read #WhiteCoatsForBlackLives. The accompanying caption stated:

> BLACK LIVES MATTER! The UF College of Medicine Office of Admissions unequivocally condemns racism, injustice, and prejudice in all forms. We acknowledge the existence and persistence of systemic oppression and racism that endanger the lives of people of color. We strive for an admissions culture that is reflective, informed and inclusive, dedicated to building a diverse community of future physicians who share a commitment to excellence and equity in healthcare.[97]

An earlier version of this page went on to say, "Please do not further burden your Black friends and colleagues by asking them to expend the

---

[97] "Medical Admissions," UF College of Medicine, https://admissions.med.ufl.edu/, accessed October 26, 2022.

energy necessary to educate you. Rather," it continued, "do the work and use existing resources to learn more on your own."

The page was later stealth-edited to remove this passage.[98] Apparently it is now okay for white and Asian University of Florida medical students to ask their black friends how they are doing.

If you check out the UFCOM admission page today, you'll find the typical image of photogenic young medical students, draped by stethoscopic necklaces, smiling at the camera. Woke rhetoric is absent.

Are these simply surface changes? It's too early to tell. *The Alligator,* an independent newspaper reporting on the University of Florida, noted in the spring 2024 semester that the first wave of changes since the state defunded DEI in public universities included closing the Office of the Chief Diversity Officer, ending DEI-focused contracts with outside vendors, and terminating thirteen full-time DEI positions. However, the paper also noted that most of the deans whose job titles once included "diversity," "equity," or "inclusion" have simply picked less hot-button words. "For example, the former associate dean for diversity, inclusion and global affairs at the College of Nursing is now the associate dean for community engagement and global affairs."[99]

Meanwhile, the associate dean for diversity and health equity in the College of Medicine became the associate dean for healthcare excellence, community, and belonging. In her former position she had declared:

> What we know is that, especially for Black, Latinx and
> Native American populations, even when you control
> for things like income, insurance and education, there
> are still disparities in patient outcomes. Research shows

---

[98] "More wokeness at the University of Florida," Do No Harm, October 13, 2022.
[99] Zoey Thomas, "UF eliminates diversity: What's known and what remains unclear," *The Alligator,* March 4, 2024.

implicit biases among physicians account for some of these disparities.[100]

It seems exceedingly unlikely that she has changed her point of view or her mission just because her title no longer features the suddenly toxic capital letters D, E, or I.

UFCOM's Code of Ethics still includes the pledge that medical students will "Acknowledge and minimize our implicit and explicit biases as we relate to others," but the UFCOM Statement of Diversity has disappeared into the ether.[101] It had formerly stated:

> Senior leadership must publically embrace, through broad, repetitive and effective communication, a definitive and unequivocal position that diversity, inclusion, and health equity is synonymous with excellence.[102]

The five schools of medicine within the University of Texas system have also been riddled with DEI dogma and policies—and they, too, are in the process of complying with (or evading) a new Texas law that expels from the state's thirteen public academic institutions such DEI fixtures as offices, training sessions, staff, mandatory statements and loyalty oaths, and all programs and activities based on race, color, ethnicity, gender identity, or sexual orientation (unless approved by the institution's general counsel and the Texas Higher Education Coordinating Board).[103]

---

[100] Tyler Francischine, "A seat at the table: Celebration of Diversity Week promoted diversity, equity and inclusion in medicine with virtual panels, talks," *Doctor Gator*, April 12, 2021, https://news.drgator.ufl.edu/2021/04/12/, accessed October 26, 2022.

[101] "Code of ethics," UF College of Medicine Office of Student Affairs, https://osa.med.ufl.edu/policies-procedures/code-of-ethics/, accessed September 18, 2024.

[102] "Statement on diversity," UF College of Medicine, https://com-main-a2.sites.medinfo.ufl.edu/files/2013/02/Statement_on_Diversity.pdf, accessed October 27, 2022. Today the URL leads to "File or Page Not Found."

[103] Marcela Rodrigues, "5 things to know about Texas' DEI ban," *Dallas Morning News*, February 27, 2024.

Spokespeople for most of the UT schools estimated that they'd get around to compliance in the fall semester of 2024. But administrators of the website of the system's flagship, the Dell Medical School of the University of Texas, haven't quite found time for their scrubbing mission. For instance, the school lists under "Admission Criteria":

> To identify future physician leaders, we look for evidence of excellence in four areas: mission contribution, personal attributes, life experiences and academic ability.[104]

Notice that "academic ability" is at the end of that list. Not exactly reassuring for those going under a knife wielded by a Dell-trained surgeon—even though he, she, or they may have fine personal attributes.

UT's Dell Med created its own medical education model, the Leading EDGE (Essentials, Delivery, Growth, and Exploration), which has a heavy emphasis on "health systems science." Students spend less than twenty hours per week in the classroom, in favor of self-directed study, and grading is pass/fail only.

"Core competencies" of the Leading EDGE curriculum are described in language that is at best opaque woke jargon, at worst gibberish. The "Health Equity" core competency requires students to:

— Describe how current and historical perceptions of identities such as race, ethnicity, language, sex, sexual orientation, gender, age, ability, culture, socioeconomic status, geographic location, immigration status and their intersectionality lead to the unequal allocation of power and resources and create vulnerabilities that influence health outcomes.

— Describe the structures of oppression such as racism and sexism that perpetuate biased biomedical assumptions and influence differential provider treatment among diverse populations.

---

[104] "How to Apply," University of Texas at Austin Dell Medical School, https://dellmed.utexas.edu/education/how-to-apply, accessed September 18, 2024.

— Gain awareness of personal conscious and unconscious bias and recognize how interpersonal power differentials manifest in actions that perpetuate health inequities.

— Identify one's own biases and demonstrate a willingness to accept and remedy them.

— Recognize one's own power and privilege and demonstrate the ability to leverage them to promote health equity.

— Recognize how a diverse health professions workforce is associated with reduced health disparities, physician-patient concordance and promotion of care that values cultural humility.

— Advocate for inclusive interpersonal, institutional and societal practices and procedures through application of understanding the role intersectional identity plays in health inequities.[105]

One longs for English translations.

Nothing in this extensive, highly politicized, and argot-ridden nonsense will help a single Dell Medicine–trained physician diagnose or treat a patient's illness. Yet as of this writing, it remains untouched by Texas's DEI law.

The UT's John Sealy School of Medicine in Galveston requires no minimum GPA or MCAT scores to be considered for admission, explaining that "academic and nonacademic factors are of equal importance."[106] Presumably these nonacademic factors are gleaned through answers to such secondary application statements as "Describe a time when you advocated for someone whose social identity (e.g., race, gender, sex,

105 "Curriculum Core Competencies," University of Texas at Austin Dell Medical School, https://dellmed.utexas.edu/education/academics/undergraduate-medical-education/leading-edge-curriculum/core-competencies, accessed September 18, 2024.

106 "John Sealy SOM Office of Admissions & Recruitment," UTMB John Sealy School of Medicine, https://www.utmb.edu/som/admissions-information/ready-to-apply-info/admission-policies-faqs, accessed September 18, 2024.

religion, socioeconomic status, ability status, etc.) differed from yours. Explain the situation and why advocacy was necessary."[107]

The Texas public-university DEI ban has made some difference. Texas A&M, which outsiders might associate with agriculture, engineering, and its cadet squad, went whole hog for wokeism. As Christopher Rufo wrote, "Texas A&M is a systematically racist institution. According to whom? According to the leadership of Texas A&M."[108] The school has engaged in public acts of self-denunciation that rival those once seen in Cuba and other communist nations.

Texas A&M College of Medicine was a leading spear of the DEI charge. Its Office of Diversity, Equity, and Inclusion promoted the usual suspects (Ibram X. Kendi, Black Lives Matter, and such videos as "Systemic Racism Explained"), and College of Medicine functionaries actually boasted to the compilers of the AAMC's Diversity, Inclusion, Culture, and Equity (DICE) Inventory of "the removal of the predominantly white male photos of graduating class [prominently] displayed on the entrance to the COM. This historic legacy now stored electronically and is available for anyone to view. We also removed the artwork honoring Dr Sims (of the Sims' speculum)."[109]

The canceled Dr. Sims was Dr. J. Marion Sims, inventor of the Sims Speculum, which is used to examine the vagina and cervix. Dr. Sims was a controversial figure, sometimes cited as the Father of Gynecology, who has been praised as a pioneer in the medical treatment of women and damned for possibly not receiving consent from some of the enslaved women upon whom he operated. He was a decidedly mixed bag, to be sure—but his invention has been a boon, even a godsend, to generations of women and their doctors.

---

[107] "University of Texas Medical Branch School of Medicine Secondary Questions," ProspectiveDoctor, https://www.prospectivedoctor.com/university-of-texas-medical-branch-school-of-medicine, accessed September 18, 2024.

[108] Christopher F. Rufo, "DEI Swallows Texas A&M," https://christopherrufo.com/, May 11, 2023.

[109] "DICE Inventory Survey," TAMU College of Medicine.

Texas A&M's current crop of bureaucrats, who have invented nothing, brag that they have canceled Dr. Sims.

However, Texas A&M College of Medicine's Office of Diversity, Equity, and Inclusion is no more, and the same is true of its counterparts across the UT system. For instance, the Texas Tech University Health Sciences Center Office of Diversity, Equity & Inclusion lives on only in not-so-fond memories and in the archives of Do No Harm, where one may read of its pushing the Gender Unicorn and ze-zie-hir pronouns on students, faculty, and staff at an institution which they vowed to hold accountable on DEI matters.[110]

Tennessee, like Texas, is fighting back against DEI tyranny.

In 2023, legislators in the Volunteer State passed and Governor Bill Lee signed the Tennessee Higher Education Freedom of Expression and Transparency Act, which was a good start at rolling back divisive diversity, equity, and inclusion requirements at publicly funded colleges and universities, including medical schools. Its key provisions include:

No DEI Statements: Applicants for employment and admission cannot be required to submit DEI statements, which medical schools increasingly use to weed out candidates who don't walk the woke party line. This helps ensure that students and faculty are chosen by merit, not politics. Getting rid of these statements creates the possibility of a more intellectually diverse campus environment, where students and their teachers are open to exploring new research ideas.

No DEI Spending: Tennessee's medical schools are prohibited from using state funds for fees, dues, subscriptions, or travel relating to an organization that requires an individual to endorse or promote a divisive concept—for example, that a certain race or sex is inherently superior to another or that the United States is fundamentally racist or sexist. This ban covers essentially every medical association and puts pressure

---

[110]   Laura L. Morgan, "The Progressive Takeover of Texas Medical Education," Do No Harm, January 2023.

on groups like the AMA and AAMC to drop their increasingly discriminatory demands.

Other victories in this Do No Harm–supported bill include welcoming campus speakers with differing views, banning discrimination against student groups based on their ideologies, requiring DEI officers to focus on workforce training and promote intellectual diversity, and notifying students and teachers of their rights, among others.

This is not to say that Tennessee's public medical schools have been cleansed of DEI. The state-funded University of Tennessee Health Science Center College of Medicine's strategic plan for 2020–2025 uses the word "diversity" twenty-nine times in a thirty-one-page document. The magic word is behind proposals to match scholarships "offered by other schools that lure our diversity applicants away"; use holistic admissions metrics to ensure student diversity; hold "racism/social justice discussions"; and develop strategies to recruit and retain a diverse faculty.[111]

And students at any of the UT Health Science Center's four locations are eligible for the Elise C. Moore Scholarship. "[P]referred recipients will be active members of the Black Student Association," says the website, though the UTHSC avoids legal scrutiny of the scholarship by adding that the Black Student Association "is interdisciplinary and open to all UTHSC students regardless of ethnic background, discipline or other affiliation."[112]

Sure.

Fed up with wokeness, Oklahoma State Superintendent Ryan Walters demanded in January 2023 that the Oklahoma State Regents for Higher Education "provide a full outline and review of every dollar"

---

[111] "College of Medicine Strategic Plan, 2020-2025," UTHSC College of Medicine, https://uthsc.edu/medicine/documents/com-strategic-plan, accessed September 19, 2024.

[112] "Elise C. Moore Scholarship," University of Tennessee Health Science Center, https://www.uthsc.edu/bsa/moore-scholarship.php, accessed September 19, 2024.

spent on DEI over the previous ten years within the Sooner State's system of twenty-five public colleges and universities.[113]

While much of the controversy had been generated by events such as a drag queen story hour for children as young as two at Oklahoma State University, Oklahoma's medical schools had embraced DEI and identity politics ideology so thoroughly as to be indistinguishable from schools in the deepest blue states.[114]

For instance, a Do No Harm investigation revealed that the University of Oklahoma College of Medicine has a department fully dedicated to advancing DEI within the institution, with frequent communication to faculty, staff, and students alike. This permanent bureaucracy pushes divisive ideas on everyone, taking time and resources away from real medical education.

The OU medical school also hires and promotes faculty based on their work on DEI. This political litmus test has nothing to do with medicine—but everything to do with ideological enforcement. Needless to say—though in the current climate it cannot be said too often—faculty should be hired not for their political views but based on their ability to teach and research at the highest level.

The OU-Tulsa School of Community Medicine offered a course and stipend that were only available to students of particular races, with whites barred. Do No Harm filed a civil rights complaint with the federal government against this rank discrimination, and Tulsa dropped the offending restriction. We also asked the feds to investigate twelve schools—including Oklahoma State University and the University of Tulsa—that participate in a recruitment program based solely on race. As I write, these cases are under review.

There is a virtue-signaling sideshow quality to some aspects of the woke spectacle in medical schools, but the entrenched DEI offices are

---

[113] "Ryan Walters' Jan. 23 request to OK Higher Education Chancellor Allison Garrett," *Tulsa World*, January 24, 2023.

[114] Shelby Kearns, "Oklahoma official demands to know 'every dollar' public universities spend on DEI," *Campus Reform*, January 30, 2023.

made up of bureaucratically minded dogmatists, and you don't want to get on their bad side. Combine ample resources with a fanatical drive to politicize all aspects of life and you've got trouble.

Much of this is beyond parody.

The Geffen School of Medicine at UCLA mandates that first-years take "Structural Racism and Health Equity," a three-to-four-hour biweekly course which includes a section in which students engage in "racial caucusing." That is, they are separated into racial groups in order to "provide a reflective space for us to explore how our positionality— particularly our racial identities as perceived within clinical spaces— influence our interaction with patients, colleagues and other staff."

This is gobbledygook. It is also a blatant violation of the 1964 Civil Rights Act, which UCLA is subject to due to its acceptance of federal monies. The course forces students to join either the "white student caucus group," the "Non-Black People of Color (NBPOC) student caucus group," or the "Black student caucus group." Students with a subversive or mischief-making bent are sternly instructed against any display of independence: they must "identify the group in which you feel you are most perceived as in clinical spaces."

Students felt powerless to challenge this racist nonsense. As one anonymous aspiring physician said, she "went to school to learn medicine, not to be segregated by the color of my skin."

Do No Harm has taken up arms against this rank bigotry, lodging a complaint with the federal Office for Civil Rights that UCLA's racial caucusing "illegally segregate[s] and separate[s] its first-year medical students based on their race, color and/or national origin."

As if segregating students by race isn't bad enough, the mandatory "Structural Racism and Health Equity" class peddles dangerous quackery to the first-years. Assigned readings for the class include an essay by "fat liberationist" Marquisele Mercedes, who says that "fatphobia is medicine's status quo" and weight loss is a "hopeless endeavor."

The syllabus for this course reads like a put-on of woke far-leftism written by an over-the-top conservative critic. Surely a medical school wouldn't force upon its new students readings that assert the evil of "ableist heteropatriarchal capitalism," refuse to spell out the word obesity (because it is a slur "used to exact violence on fat people"), and celebrate "gender self-determination" with no reference to the wholesale rethinking of the wisdom of childhood transitioning that is roiling the waters in Europe! Sadly, the Geffen School does.

The invaluable investigative reporter Aaron Sibarium of the *Washington Free Beacon* has covered and uncovered the scandal at UCLA.

Jeffrey Flier, former dean of Harvard Medical School (2007–2016) and a major figure in the study of obesity and diabetes, told Sibarium that the UCLA curriculum "promotes extensive and dangerous misinformation." The med school, Dr. Flier said, "has centered this required course on a socialist/Marxist ideology that is totally inappropriate. As a longstanding medical educator, I found this course truly shocking."

He continued, "This is a profoundly misguided view of obesity, a complex medical disorder with major adverse health consequences for all racial and ethnic groups. Promotion of these ignorant ideas to medical students without counterbalancing input from medical experts in the area is nothing less than pedagogical malpractice."

As if flaunting its utter madness, the mandatory "Structural Racism and Health Equity" course has also featured a pro-Hamas activist who goes by the name Lisa Gray-Garcia. This nutjob ordered the future doctors to put their fists to the floor and pray to "Mama Earth." They were also instructed to chant "Free, Free Palestine."[115] Many of the young people I speak to shrug at this kind of ridiculousness, but they are powerless to stop it.

---

[115] Aaron Sibarium, "UCLA Med School Requires Students To Attend Lecture Where Speaker Demands Prayer for 'Mama Earth,' Leads Chants of 'Free Palestine,'" *Washington Free Beacon*, April 2, 2024.

The contempt with which DEI propagandists view those who have the audacity to disagree was recently on display at Washington University School of Medicine in St. Louis.

Kaytlin Reedy-Rogier, lecturer and coleader of Wash U's "Understanding Systemic Racism" team, was filmed by a camera-wielding med student warning her class that "if you try to fight me or debate me" on the matter of systemic racism, "I will shut that shit down real fast."[116]

This is not exactly in the Voltairean "I may disagree with what you say but I will defend to the death your right to say it" tradition.

Reedy-Rogier was speaking to a class in "Health Equity & Justice," which is part of the med school's mandatory "Gateway Curriculum." It's easy to snicker at this cartoonish tough guy/gal intolerance, but this is also tremendously sad. Washington University of St. Louis is one of the outstanding research institutions in the country. Yet it is undermining that legacy with a racist approach to medical education.

While not every lecturer is as brutally honest about his or her bias as Ms. Reedy-Rogier, the unfortunate fact is that of the top fifty medical schools, thirty-nine impose mandatory student training or coursework in DEI, critical race theory, anti-racism, implicit bias, or cultural competency.[117]

At the University of Minnesota Medical School, new students participating in the venerable ritual of the white coat ceremony recite a grotesque burlesque of the Hippocratic Oath in which they pledge fealty to every ort and speck of woke nonsense. Just for starters, the aspiring doctors are forced to recite, like browbeaten POWs:

> *We commit to uprooting the legacy and perpetuation of structural violence deeply embedded within the health care system.*

116 Emma Colton, "Washington U lecturer warns medical students not to 'debate' her on 'systemic oppression': 'shut that' down," Fox News, December 18, 2022.
117 "Our Top 50 Medical School Database," Critical Race Training in Education, https://criticalrace.org/.

We recognize inequities built by past and present traumas rooted in white supremacy, colonialism, the gender binary, ableism, and all forms of oppression.

As we enter this profession with opportunity for growth, we commit to promoting a culture of antiracism, listening, and amplifying voices for positive change.

We pledge to honor all indigenous ways of healing that have been historically marginalized by western medicine.

It goes on and on, in a similar vein.

Reciting the new pledge along with associate dean Dr. Robert Englander, the students must forget about the traditional role of the physician as a healer of the sick and instead express guilt for the incredible advances in medicine that have enabled huge improvements in longevity and freedom from some of the most devastating childhood diseases. They must fight "the gender binary, white supremacy, and colonialism" rather than illness and disease. "Heal the sick" is subordinated to honoring "all indigenous ways of healing that have been historically marginalized by Western medicine."

Does Dean Englander mean that we should embrace shamanism?

Probably not. But then as the heroic anti–critical race theory scholar Christopher Rufo remarked upon viewing a recording of this spectacle, "The most incredible thing about this clip is that the doctor almost certainly doesn't believe in what he's saying. But he submits anyway— because the institutional powers now require otherwise intelligent people to falsify their own beliefs and repeat the left-wing copypasta."[118]

---

[118] Breccan F. Thies, "Minnesota Medical Students Swear Oath to Fight 'White Supremacy,' 'Honor All Indigenous Ways of Healing,'" *Breitbart*, October 13, 2022.

- - - - - -

Although it will take time to see how institutions of higher education respond to the US Supreme Court's ruling in *Students for Fair Admissions v. Harvard* and *Students for Fair Admissions v. UNC*, a freshet of lawsuits is about to rush over the med-school admissions landscape. In striking down discriminatory treatment of college applicants on the basis of race, the court spoke in pellucidly clear language, not open to pettifogging or quibbling: "Distinctions between citizens solely because of their ancestry are by their very nature odious to a free people whose institutions are founded upon the doctrine of equality." This means no discrimination based on race. Period. "Eliminating racial discrimination means eliminating all of it," said the court.[119]

The decisions provoked an immediate reaction from the usual suspects that might have been scripted by a middling AI service. Dr. David J. Skorton, AAMC president, and Frank Trinity, AAMC chief legal officer, pronounced themselves "deeply disappointed." The court, they charged, had demonstrated "a lack of understanding of the critical benefits of racial and ethnic diversity in educational settings and a failure to recognize the urgent need to address health inequities in our country."

By contrast, these sages of AAMC, "informed by decades of research"—which they fail to cite—recognized "the undeniable benefits of diversity for improving the health of people everywhere." As if asserting a truism so obvious that no evidence in its support need be adduced, the AAMC duo stated that "a diverse and inclusive biomedical research workforce with individuals from historically excluded and underrepresented groups in biomedical research is critical to gathering the range of perspectives needed to identify and solve the complex scientific problems of today and tomorrow."[120]

---

[119]   *Students for Fair Admissions, Inc. v. Harvard* (2023) 600 U.S. 181.
[120]   David J. Skorton and Frank Trinity, "AAMC Deeply Disappointed by SCOTUS Decision on Race-Conscious Admissions," press release, June 29, 2023.

No sooner had the court handed down its Solomonic ruling than AAMC officials were plotting end-runs around it. After all, as president Skorton explained, "Lives depend on us diversifying the health care workforce."

Sure, schools may no longer use race as a factor in whether to admit an applicant, but there's more than one way to skin this cat. Leila Amiri, associate dean of admissions at Larner College of Medicine at the University of Vermont, explained to AAMCNews that while "race in and of itself" could no longer be used as a "measure of diversity," an applicant's "experiences" could be. Those dots just beg to be connected.

AAMC officials note that "holistic review," which usually includes a personal interview—wink, wink—remains permissible, and so do essays, which "might include experiences or perspectives related to the applicant's race." In other words, race will remain a consideration, though schools won't be so openly discriminatory.[121]

Yet if institutions seek quotas and DEI by furtive means, well-qualified whites or Asians who were rejected by medical schools or residencies will file suit. In fact, Do No Harm is currently looking for young men and women who have been unfairly rejected for medical school admission and residencies.

Any kid who attaches his name to such a lawsuit is going to be plastered with a scarlet letter and crucified on social media. The virulence and hatred of the cancel-culture cult makes many people understandably reluctant to be publicly identified with anti-DEI efforts. But the *Harvard* ruling points the way forward. Those bringing the suits did not name individual plaintiffs. This anonymity protects an injured party from vengeful nutcases and antifa thugs. The plaintiff in the cases we file will be Do No Harm; in effect, the anonymous member's standing will transfer to the organization.

121   Patrick Boyle, "How can medical schools boost racial diversity in the wake of the recent Supreme Court ruling?" AAMCNews, July 27, 2023.

To date, the courts are divided over whether a person who believes that under law he should be eligible for a program but who does not want his name made public may sue. Case law is conflicted on this matter, so the anonymity question may be decided by the US Supreme Court. When it is, we are optimistic that we'll be on the winning side.

CHAPTER FIVE

IMPLICIT BIAS/EXPLICIT DISCRIMINATION

There is no credible evidence that physicians are biased, or healthcare is systematically racist. The psychological test that is commonly used to prove such claims, the Implicit Association Test, has been thoroughly repudiated. Even its creators have acknowledged its shortcomings.

I don't mean to suggest that there is no such thing as implicit bias. I think it is a real phenomenon. Daniel Kahneman won a Nobel Prize in Economics for his work in behavior science, including cognitive biases, which he popularized in *Thinking, Fast and Slow* (2011). But the relevant question for medicine is: Does implicit bias influence behavior?

The Implicit Association Test (IAT), which you can take for free online at a website hosted by Harvard University (https://implicit.harvard.edu/implicit) was unveiled by University of Washington researchers in 1998 and lifted on a manufactured wave of publicity into the realm of paradigm-shifting discoveries on the order of the telescope or penicillin.

Do I exaggerate? Consider the words of Harvard psychologist Mahzarin Banaji, an implicit bias cofounder and popularizer:

> [It] will challenge our beliefs about the very nature of our own minds.... [I]t is not merely about the place of our planet amongst other planets, it's not merely about our place in the larger set of other species, it's about the core issue of our competence, it's about our goodness, our ability to be moral, and to have control over our thoughts and feelings, about the most important object in our universe, other humans.

Whew!

This test, which supposedly measures the "unconscious racism" that, we are encouraged to believe, motivates racist behavior by physicians and others, was boosted by a sales job that would have made Elizabeth Anne "Theranos" Holmes proud.

The IAT works like this:

Images appear on a screen, and you press a button as soon as they come up. Perhaps a white man and the word "good" appear first; you press the button as soon as this registers in your mind. Then a picture of a black man and the word "good" appears; again, you press the button. If you take a millisecond more to press the black man's button you are said to be biased against him. Other words—ugly, handsome, etc.—follow, as do images, and you keep pressing buttons.

Now, it turns out that there may be several reasons for this lag of a millisecond in your different reactions to pictures of black and white people and various words. Perhaps you believe that black people have been treated poorly for generations, so you hesitate oh so briefly. This feeling of sympathy will be interpreted as bias. Other factors that muddle test results include "knowing the purpose of the test, faking the test results, repeatedly taking the test, being in the presence of African

Americans, cognitive quickness and flexibility, physical speed, and manual dexterity."[122]

The test is one giant "gotcha!" You don't feel racist, but IAT reveals that deep down you *are* racist. You—and up to 95 percent of your countrymen and women—exhibit the "roots of unconscious prejudice."

Even its designers admit that the IAT is unreliable. Its findings are not reproducible. If you take the test at an interval of two weeks, you'll get a different result about half the time. Since 80 percent reproducibility is the usual threshold, the IAT's 55 percent reliability mark is not nearly good enough. The test floats in a sea of false positives and false negatives. In fact, there is not *"any* published evidence that the race IAT has test-retest reliability that is close to acceptable for real-world evaluation. If you take the test today, and then take it again tomorrow—or even in just a few hours—there's a solid chance you'll get a very different result." (Italics in original) Yet as Jesse Singal wrote in a powerfully debunking piece in *New York* magazine, "the IAT went viral not for solid scientific reasons, but simply because it tells us such a simple, pat story about how racism works and can be fixed: that deep down, we're all a little—or a lot—racist, and that if we measure and study this individual-level racism enough, progress toward equality will ensue."

On top of the IAT's weak reproducibility, there is no solid evidence connecting its results with behavior. Just because someone hesitates for a fraction of a second in pressing the correct button does not mean that person discriminates against black people in his or her daily life. The architects of the test have admitted that "attempts to diagnostically use such measures for individuals risk undesirably high rates of erroneous classifications."

Okay—an individual's test results tell us nothing about his prejudice (or lack thereof) and its connection to his behavior. It does not translate to the real world.

---

122 Althea Nagai, "The Implicit Association Test: Flawed Science Tricks Americans into Believing They Are Unconscious Racists," Heritage Foundation, December 12, 2017.

So what practical good is it?

The handful of papers asserting a link between test results and behavior are riddled with "serious methodological problems" that range all the way up to fabricated evidence (which was blamed on an "overzealous undergraduate").[123]

In a research paper for the Heritage Foundation, Dr. Althea Nagai pointed to the adoption of the IAT by medical schools:

> Prompted by the Association of American Medical Colleges' concern with diversity and unconscious bias, medical schools such as Stanford, Ohio State, and Johns Hopkins encourage faculty and students to take the IAT, declaring the test to be both reliable and valid, ignoring its controversy in psychology and related social sciences. Duke University has gone one step further and incorporated it into a second-year medical school course on unconscious bias.[124]

Unreliable as IAT is, it is no parlor game or idle time-waster. It has been weaponized. Dr. Quinn Capers, former associate dean of admissions and vice dean of faculty affairs at The Ohio State University College of Medicine, and his colleagues Dr. Daniel Clinchot, OSUCOM's vice dean for education, and Dr. Leon McDougle, chief diversity officer, are on record claiming that "implicit white race preference has been associated with discrimination in the education, criminal justice, and health care systems and could impede the entry of African Americans into the medical profession, where they and other minorities remain underrepresented." To address this alleged problem, OSUCOM inflicts the IAT on faculty members and members of the admissions committee.[125]

---

[123] Jesse Singal, "Psychology's Favorite Tool for Measuring Racism Isn't Up to the Job," *New York*, January 11, 2017.

[124] Althea Nagai, "The Implicit Association Test."

[125] Quinn Capers et al., "Implicit racial bias in medical school admissions," *Academic Medicine* 92, no. 3 (March 2017): 365–369.

Dr. Capers reported—with great satisfaction, one imagines—"significant levels of implicit or unconscious preference for certain racial and gender groups." He used this data to develop the OSUCOM implicit bias training course.[126]

Thanks to academic administrators like Dr. Capers, an entire edifice of indoctrination and ideological browbeating has been erected on the flimsy foundation of the IAT.

- - - - - -

DEI advocates point to bias whenever racial disparities are observed in medical treatment.

For instance, the *Philadelphia Inquirer* made hay of a study showing that minority kids have their blood sugar level controlled less well than white kids. The article was based on an editorial in the medical journal *Pediatrics* by two pediatric endocrinologists at Children's Hospital of Philadelphia alleging that the reason minority kids have less access to insulin pumps is medical racism.[127]

I went back and read the study upon which this editorial was based. It used three databases: one in Germany, Switzerland, and Austria; one in Australia and New Zealand; and one in the United States. In each database, including those whose countries had no history of slavery or sizeable black population, the blood sugar level was less well-controlled in minority children with Type 1 diabetes than in others.[128]

I followed the paper trail of citations back to the original source, which was a survey of US pediatric endocrinologists that asked if race made a difference in whether or not they used an insulin pump with a child. The answer they gave? No. Instead, the reason black kids used

---

[126] "Implicit Bias Training," The Ohio State University College of Medicine, https://medicine.osu.edu/diversity/initiatives/implicit-bias-training, accessed June 12, 2023.
[127] Colin P. Hawkes and Terri H. Lipman, "Racial Disparities in Pediatric Type 1 Diabetes: Yet Another Consequence of Structural Racism," *Pediatrics* 148, no. 2 (August 2021).
[128] Jennifer L. Sherr et al., "Hemoglobin A1c Patterns of Youth With Type 1 Diabetes 10 Years Post Diagnosis From 3 Continents," *Pediatrics* 148, no. 2 (2021).

insulin pumps less often had to do with insurance status. These families were likelier to be on Medicaid, which imposes considerable burdens. If the child is to get an insulin pump, for instance, his or her blood sugar has to be measured and recorded three times a day. If mom is working and dad is not in the home, this is impossible to do. So the doctors put the kids on three insulin shots a day, a regimen which *does not* require rigorous measurement.

This whole insulin-pump racism story was a house of cards. It was based on a false narrative by a reporter with an agenda. That's what you find with implicit bias claims. There's just no evidence for them. Every time you see one of these stories it turns out that you can explain 80–90 percent of the difference in healthcare outcomes using the accepted parameters. But you can't get at that other 10 percent. There's always some uncertainty left, which they attribute to bias.

What they never attribute these disparities to is *patient behavior*. If a family of whatever race, color, or creed does not take a child to the pediatrician, whether due to neglect or laziness or drug abuse or lack of transportation, pediatric medicine cannot be blamed. The way to close at least part of the health-outcomes gap is by better outreach to the community, more effective education, reforms to the health insurance system, and similar concrete measures.

- - - - - -

The kidney societies are into a masochistic form of self-abasement. They have declared themselves racist, and by implication they have slandered past generations of nephrologists as monsters who by their conscious or unconscious racism delivered poorer care to black patients than to non-black patients, which is the only explanation they will countenance for the disparity in black/non-black kidney disease outcomes.

With a shockingly cavalier dismissal of alternative possibilities, they say that black patients have been shortchanged in the receipt of kidney transplants because white physicians discriminate against them.

This is both offensive and a lie. For one thing, the only entity that has an economic incentive to discourage transplants is the dialysis industry, which loses customers every time someone gains a kidney. But the relevant physicians are not employed by dialysis companies.

The reason black patients are less likely to receive a kidney transplant than similarly afflicted non-blacks is that many don't want them. They don't trust the system, so they are less likely to go for evaluations. Many poor patients who have low health literacy do not adhere to the prescribed medical regimens, and doctors know that such patients, who often do not take their immunosuppressant drugs, will lose their kidneys. In fact, studies show that black transplant recipients lose their kidneys much more quickly than whites do.[129]

There are solid reasons why doctors hesitate to send what they believe to be unreliable patients, of whatever race, color, creed, or sex, for transplants. If they do not strictly adhere to the regimen it's going to be a mess. They will die or at least lose their transplanted kidneys to immune rejection.

Put simply, blacks get proportionately fewer kidney transplants than non-blacks because they are disproportionately poor, disproportionately nonadherent to the regimen for transplant patients, and may have genetic variants that predispose them to kidney failure. There is nothing racist about this, unless you think every statistical difference between blacks and non-blacks, from the racial breakdown of birdwatchers to the racial breakdown of NFL cornerbacks, is due to racism.

Yet the kidney societies persist in self-flagellation. One way to get on the transplant list is to have a certain level of decrement of kidney function. The measurement of kidney function had been very imprecise until in 1999 Andrew Levey, a nephrologist at Tufts University, came up with a formula to gauge how effectively the kidney is filtering blood. He refined this significant medical breakthrough in 2009.

---

[129] David J. Taber et al., "Twenty years of evolving trends in racial disparities for adult kidney transplant recipients," *Kidney International* 90, no. 4 (October 2016): 878–887.

This formula reliably estimates the decrement that would be found by a radioactive tracer—except for black patients, who because of differences in muscle mass and an associated blood factor used to measure kidney function received inaccurate results. So the scores of black patients were adjusted with a correction factor that more accurately revealed their actual decrement of function.

The disputed correction factor, which increased the scores of black patients, was decried as a tool of white supremacy and a way to make black people seem healthier than they really were, which lessened their chance of being placed on the transplant list. Never mind that the real effect of the correction factor was to more precisely estimate the decrement of function level—it had to be canceled. And it was.

In the *Wall Street Journal*, Sam Cox nicely laid out the issue:

> Nephrology is under fire from the left for including race as a factor in the assessment of renal function. Large, cross-sectional studies assessing kidney function in relation to several variables repeatedly found strong correlations between self-identification as "black" and certain variations in normal kidney function. Their authors saw fit to include blackness in their standardized equations, now commonly used in the assessment of renal function.
>
> Subsequent backlash from woke physicians, contending that race as a "social construct" ought not be considered in diagnosis, led to the re-evaluation of these equations. New studies demonstrate the tragic consequences of removing the "black" variable: inappropriate dosage of chemotherapeutics, rejection of potential kidney donors and exclusion from clinical trials. Paradoxically, the fight to remove race from the equation goes

on, at cross-purposes with the well-being of the black community.[130]

Rather than race, maybe we should take ideology out of the equation?

If only...

Mathematician Paul Williams, biostatistician at the prestigious Lawrence Livermore National Laboratory and a fellow of Do No Harm, has studied and written carefully on this subject. Paul concludes that "a strong case can be made for retaining the race-corrected 2009 CKD-EPI formula," but the apposite medical journals will not publish his papers.

Paul is beside himself. He knows what's going on. Scrapping Dr. Levey's formula in favor of the new woke one is a gross episode of intellectual dishonesty that will have deleterious consequences for non-black kidney patients without benefiting black kidney patients.

In knee-jerk fashion, the National Kidney Foundation and the American Society of Nephrology Task Force on Reassessing the Inclusion of Race in Diagnosing Kidney Disease junked the 2009 race-corrected CKD (chronic kidney disease) formula and advocated the adoption of the race-free formula by nephrologists and laboratories. The projected effect, wrote Williams, was to "negate CKD in 5.51 million White and other non-Black adults and reclassify CKD to less severe stages in another 4.59 million non-Blacks, in order to expand treatment eligibility to 434,000 Blacks not previously diagnosed and to 584,000 Blacks previously diagnosed with less severe CKD."[131]

Ten million white, Asian, Hispanic, and other patients were thereby downgraded or disqualified for kidney treatment eligibility. In terms of

[130] Letters, "How a Hospital Thinks About Systemic Racism," *Wall Street Journal*, May 2, 2022.

[131] Paul Williams, "Retaining Race in Chronic Kidney Disease Diagnosis and Treatment," *Cureus* 15, no. 9 (September 2023): e45054. Figures taken from James A. Diao, Andrew S. Levey, et al., "National Projections for Clinical Implications of Race-Free Creatine-Based GFR Estimating Equations," *Journal of the American Society of Nephrology* 34, no. 2 (February 2023): 309–321.

real life (and death) this translates to chronic kidney disease sufferers having their transplants delayed—and possibly dying before going under the knife—while black patients with less severe CKD receive treatment that they may not have needed.

The nephrology societies know that condemnation of Dr. Levey's decrement-of-function formula is nonsense, but they went along with it, because they feared being called racist by woke fanatics more than they valued truth and the lives of those who were pushed down the list for the crime of being non-black.

The extent to which this reign of terror and intimidation holds sway can be seen in the example of the renal-function formula's lead developer. When it first came under attack, Dr. Levey defended it, saying that while he welcomed the consideration of rival measurements, this was the best formula he could come up with.

But soon enough he abandoned ship, coauthoring a paper that supported throwing out his formula for the new, less accurate one. He and his coauthors explained that their "choice is consistent with a core value of the NKF-ASN Task Force to promote equity, as opposed to equality, in kidney health."[132] After all, nobody wants to be smeared as a racist, much less the designer of an allegedly racist measurement.

Dissenters from DEI-skewed medicine are denigrated and ostracized. The scientific method, which enjoins testing and retesting and modifying hypotheses, seems not to apply when the issue of race touches upon a scientific question.

Perhaps it is because of my background, but I am acutely aware of the cowardice and downright malevolence that are driving the racialization of nephrology.

In mid-2024, the DEI-driven bureaucrats at the Centers for Medicare & Medicaid Services proposed a rule change to the Increasing Organ Transplant Access (IOTA) Model that would incentivize hospitals

---

[132]   Williams, "Retaining Race."

to create so-called "health equity" goals to reduce disparities in treatment for end-stage renal disease (ESRD).

As is usually the case, the verbiage seemed benign and beyond dispute. Who is against increasing access to organ transplants? Who supports health *in*equity? Yet under this rule, providers would almost certainly and intentionally select patients for kidney transplantation based on race.

The CMS proposal mandated that participating kidney hospitals submit so-called health-equity plans. The language was vague—purposely so—and did not preclude, let alone discourage, participating hospitals from giving patients of certain racial communities priority over others. Participating hospitals must set "health equity goals" or "targeted outcomes," and it is difficult to conceive how this would not lead to some, most, or all hospitals reaching these goals through race-based ends.

The rule would almost certainly—and intentionally—result in the selection of patients with end-stage renal disease for kidney transplantation based on race. Given that only about 31 percent of patients with ESRD receive transplants, this rule would run afoul of *Students for Fair Admissions v. Harvard*, in which the US Supreme Court observed that "[a] benefit provided to some...but not others necessarily advantages the former group at the expense of the latter."[133] Organ transplantation is a zero-sum game. Some patients will be deprived of transplantation, which CMS acknowledges as the "best treatment for" ESRD, because of irrelevant factors like the color of their skin.[134]

A more sensible solution—one focused on patient education—is possible and advisable. For example, the authors of one study on racial disparities in kidney transplantation wrote:

> From the beginning of the transplant-seeking process,
> our study found that blacks began transplant evaluation

---

[133] *Students for Fair Admissions, Inc. v. Harvard* (2023) 600 U.S. 181.
[134] "Medicare Program; Alternative Payment Model Updates and the Increasing Organ Transplant Access (IOTA) Model," 89 *Fed. Reg.* 43,518 (May 17, 2024).

less willing to get on the deceased donor waitlist, less willing for LDKT (living donor kidney transplantation), and less knowledgeable about the benefits of transplant compared with whites. As patients moved through the transplant process, those patients with less transplant knowledge and motivation to pursue LDKT at transplant onset were ultimately less likely to complete evaluation or receive LDKTs years later. When patients' initial knowledge and attitudinal differences were controlled in the multivariable modeling, the racial disparity in receipt of LDKTs disappeared.[135]

A patient's willingness to endure the rigors of transplantation should be decisive, not a patient's race.

Consistent with our goal of protecting healthcare from identity politics, Do No Harm immediately took up arms against this proposed rule, which encouraged providers to limit access to and availability of healthcare services on the basis of race. This certainly includes organ transplants, which are often lifesaving, and which may be the best treatment for the more than eight hundred thousand Americans with end-stage renal disease.

To that end, I submitted a comment to CMS Administrator Chiquita Brooks-LaSure opposing this iniquitous plan to favor some racial groups in the kidney-transplant process over others. I told her that as a matter of policy, law, and morality, this cannot stand.[136]

And it did not. In late November 2024, the Biden administration and CMS backed down, scrapping the health equity payment adjustment.

---

[135] Amy D. Waterman et al., "Modifiable patient characteristics and racial disparities in evaluation completion and living donor transplant," *Clinical Journal of the American Society of Nephrology* 8, no. 6 (June 2013): 995–1002.

[136] Stanley Goldfarb, Letter to Hon. Chiquita Brooks-LaSure, "Do No Harm Calls on CMS to Withdraw Proposed Rule that Encourages Racial Prioritization for Kidney Transplants," Do No Harm, June 12, 2024.

Those who advocate the resegregation of medicine marshal in their defense a fatally flawed study of maternal mortality in which investigators looked at internet photos of physicians from a Florida database and concluded that black babies had a higher survival rate as neonates if they had black doctors rather than non-black doctors.[137]

Interesting, if true. Yet the researchers did not adjust for risk. They excluded infants under 1500 grams of weight from the study. These babies had much higher death rates, and the sicker babies had disproportionately more white neonatologists. When looking at health outcomes you must consider the risk that the patient brings to the operating table.

This is a mistake on the order of asserting that because the death rate at the Hospital of the University of Pennsylvania is higher than that at Community Hospital, Community must be a better hospital. No—what's happening is that Community transfers really sick patients to Penn.

On the same misdirected track, about fifteen years ago the local Philadelphia papers published death rates for cardiac surgeons. The guy at the bottom of the heap one year was near the top of the heap the next year, not because he had miraculously honed his skills to world-class level but rather because he simply stopped taking the really tough cases.

Poorly conceived studies like the Florida one have an unfortunately long shelf life if they serve a progressive narrative.

None other than US Supreme Court Justice Ketanji Brown Jackson dragged the misconceived black-babies-need-black-doctors paper into her dissent in *Students for Fair Admissions v. Harvard*. Footnoting the Association of American Medical Colleges, she wrote, "For high-risk

---

[137] Brad N. Greenwood et al., "Physician–patient racial concordance and disparities in birthing mortality for newborns," *Proceedings of the National Academy of Sciences of the United States of America* 117, no. 35 (September 2020): 21194–21200.

Black newborns, having a Black physician more than doubles the likelihood that the baby will live, and not die."[138]

My friend Jay P. Greene, senior research fellow at the Heritage Foundation, took a cue from the racetrack and described Justice Jackson's contention as a "trifecta of wrong." Namely, "She was factually incorrect in describing the results of a study that should not be believed, which wouldn't provide practical support for her argument even if it were accurate and credible."[139]

Justice Jackson's math—or that of her clerks—is way off. As Greene notes of the Florida study, black babies with a black physician had a survival rate of 99.6839 percent, while those with a white attending physician had a survival rate of 99.5549 percent. The former number is not, to put it mildly, double that of the latter.

Moreover, as previously mentioned, seriously ill babies and those with very low birth weights were disproportionately treated by white physicians. It is expected that such infants will have a lower survival rate than healthy babies. As Jay Greene and Do No Harm's director of research Ian Kingsbury wrote, "We have many reasons to believe that the process by which doctors are assigned to newborns is not random and is instead strongly related to the likelihood that newborns will die."

Even if medical school admissions were relaxed to admit and graduate a vast increase in the number of black doctors, the resultant pairing up of physicians with expectant mothers along racial lines would "require racial segregation in health care that would run afoul of widely accepted legal and political opposition to such practices."[140] It would be a throwback to the ugly regime of racial segregation—and it would rightly offend even those with a rudimentary moral sense.

[138] Justice Jackson, dissenting, *Students for Fair Admissions, Inc. v. Harvard* (2023) 600 U.S. 181.

[139] Jay P. Greene, "Justice Jackson's Trifecta of Wrong on 'Research' on Racial Preferences," Heritage Foundation, July 10, 2023.

[140] Ian Kingsbury and Jay Greene, "Racial Concordance in Medicine: The Return of Segregation," Do No Harm, December 2023.

As Ian Kingsbury observes, "a great deal of contemporary medical literature is policy-based evidence-making" rather than the reverse. "Advocates pass off their agendas as 'science' so they can claim that their worldview is enlightened. They torture data to manipulate results, oversell findings, and mischaracterize other research in plain sight."

What is especially galling about these claims of bias is that there is absolutely no evidence that they are true. Having greater diversity in the medical field may in some respects be a desirable thing, but there is zero evidence that it improves healthcare outcomes. It's all nonsense.

Yet the nation's dominant medical institutions are changing the way that people are recruited into healthcare and educated for healthcare careers on the basis of this arrant fallacy. And they are spending a fortune on this fool's errand!

Do No Harm recognizes the disparities in healthcare outcomes among races, particularly with respect to black and Latino persons compared with whites and Asians, and we have proposed workable solutions.

The main problem is access. Black patients, especially, are less likely to show up for treatment at the early stages of disease. This has been tirelessly documented.

For instance, a recent study of the increasing prevalence of uterine cancer found that on average, black women show up eight months after the first symptoms of abnormal bleeding, while for white women the average is three months. That gap is one reason that black women are almost twice as likely to die from this form of cancer than are white women.[141]

No doctor, upon meeting a black woman who reports abdominal bleeding, says, "You're black. I'm not going to treat you." What does happen is that treatment requires informed consent, and patients who lack trust in doctors or are less health literate are likelier to withhold that

---

[141] Brianna Abbott, "Uterine Cancer Was Easy to Treat. Now It's Killing More Women Than Ever," *Wall Street Journal*, February 12, 2024.

consent. They have agency, but they are not using it properly. Thus the discrepancy in the utilization of services.

It has to do with education, not racist doctors. The solution offered by the DEI crowd—force doctors to take implicit bias training—is worse than useless. It treats a nonexistent problem and only breeds resentment in doctors who are accused of nonexistent bias.

Forcing someone to sit through a lecture in which their racial or ethnic group is targeted as the locus of evil in the world is demeaning, insulting, dishonest, and has no place in a free country.

Even the *Chronicle of Higher Education*, which uncritically regurgitates DEI talking points, had to admit that DEI training is often counterproductive. In its 2024 report "The Future of Diversity Training: Better Ways to Make Your College More Inclusive," the *Chronicle* reports that 47 percent of survey participants find such training at best "neither helpful nor unhelpful," and at worst, "very/somewhat unhelpful."

The report goes on to say:

> Diversity-training programs are now practically a rite of passage for college faculty and staff members, yet the evidence that they are effective is underwhelming.... While there is a significant body of research on diversity training dating back decades, many studies rely on surveys that ask how participants felt about the training or assess what they've learned, while relatively few try to determine whether the training changed how people behave.... The studies that do exist have found mixed results. Some show that participants learn about people from other backgrounds and that training can have an effect on beliefs and behaviors (although the latter fades over time). Others show that diversity-training programs can trigger negative feelings in participants and even harm the very groups they're intended to help.

One chart from the report even suggests that certain DEI trainings actually *decrease* diversity, with a 13.9 percent drop in black female managers following diversity trainings. This is a sharper decline than experienced by any other subgroup.

Yet nothing—especially evidence—can shake the faith of the true believer.[142]

A study by the Network Contagion Research Institute and the Rutgers University Social Perception Lab, "Instructing Animosity: How DEI Pedagogy Produces the Hostile Attribution Bias," found—astonishingly and frighteningly—that those exposed to DEI training exhibited increased agreement with Adolf Hitler's rhetoric and had a greater desire to punish those they perceived as harboring prejudice, even when none existed.

In the former instance, the researchers discovered that survey participants who read DEI narratives about the Hindu caste system which took Hitler quotes and substituted the word "Brahmin" for "Jew" were "markedly more likely" than those in a control group to "endorse Hitler's demonization statements, agreeing that Brahmins are 'parasites' (+35.4%), 'viruses' (+33.8%), and 'the devil personified' (+27.1%)." The authors concluded, "These findings suggest that exposure to anti-oppressive narratives can increase the endorsement of the type of demonization and scapegoating characteristic of authoritarianism."

In the latter instance, reading the works of "anti-racist" activists Ibram X. Kendi and Robin DiAngelo actually "engendered a hostile attribution bias, amplifying perceptions of prejudicial hostility where none was present, and punitive responses to the imaginary prejudice."[143]

---

142 "The Future of Diversity Training: Better Ways to Make Your College More Inclusive," *The Chronicle of Higher Education*, 2024.

143 Ankita Jagdeep et al., "Instructing Animosity: How DEI Pedagogy Produces the Hostile Attribution Bias," Network Contagion Research Institute (NCRI) and the Rutgers University Social Perception Lab, 2024. See also "Study Finds DEI Training Increases Agreement With Hitler's Rhetoric—And the Media Won't Touch It," Do No Harm, November 25, 2024.

Feeding racial paranoia and encouraging physicians to find prejudice under every bed is a recipe for disaster. In the medical field, where patients trust healthcare professionals with their very lives, it is madness—even evil—to subject doctors and nurses to propaganda that encourages authoritarian, prejudicial impulses.

- - - - - -

Even in states with governments committed to being "woke," we don't have to sit back and take whatever propaganda or politicized tests the powers that be try to ram down our throats.

Consider Michigan, where at the direction of Governor Gretchen Whitmer as many as four hundred thousand healthcare workers in twenty-six medical fields—not only doctors and nurses, but athletic trainers, acupuncturists, massage therapists, midwives, and many others—are now required to learn about implicit bias every time they apply for or renew a license.

Michigan is one of seven states that require implicit bias training for medical professionals, and its mandate is among the most expansive in the nation. Alarmingly, at least twenty-five other states are considering a similar imposition.

Working with the Mackinac Center, a Michigan think tank, and thanks to the generous support of a donor, Do No Harm designed a course that met Governor Whitmer's criteria but did not spread the misinformation endemic to implicit bias training. It launched May 1, 2024—and it has thrown a sorely needed monkey wrench into Governor Whitmer's indoctrination scheme.

The authors of the Michigan law no doubt want every medical professional in the state to accept the woke party line on race. But Do No Harm's course goes in a more ethical—and less political—direction. Instead of teaching implicit bias as fact, we're telling medical professionals the truth: that this training is grounded in falsehood and is a direct threat to the health and well-being of patients.

How are we able to offer this course? Michigan requires providers to be "a nationally recognized or state-recognized health-related organization," which we are. We also provide "information on implicit bias," another requirement. And Do No Harm's course includes "strategies to reduce disparities in access to and delivery of health care services."

Our course starts with key facts about implicit bias, including the nature of the training that purports to combat it. As my colleague Laura Morgan has written, implicit bias training is generally filled with insulting accusations against medical professionals, including overtly racist statements and assumptions. Medical professionals have been told in training that they contribute to "modern-day lynchings in the workplace" and that their "implicit bias kills." This isn't medical education. It's ideological claptrap.

The real point of such mandates as Michigan's is to steep medical professionals in a divisive worldview. Our course exposes how such training serves an "anti-racist" agenda, which is in fact deeply racist, since "anti-racism" demands discriminatory treatment based on skin color.

Do No Harm's course also illuminates one of the most disturbing premises of wokeness in medicine. The concept of implicit bias is closely connected to the assertion that white doctors are hurting or even killing black patients, a simplistic and false argument based on the existence of real yet complicated health disparities. This argument is predicated on the belief—explicitly stated at medical schools and by major medical associations—that health outcomes improve when patients and physicians are matched by race. That's false, as our course shows with a thorough review of the scholarly evidence. More to the point, "racial concordance," as activists call it, is a thinly veiled argument for the resegregation of medicine.

The Do No Harm course is available for a minimal fee to every medical professional in Michigan. We hope it will become the default choice for new-license and renewal applicants alike. It may also meet continuing medical education requirements for medical professionals in other states (Oregon is near the top of the list), and it could be relevant for workers in non-medical industries who have been told to get training about implicit bias. Do No Harm is freeing medical professionals from woke brainwashing so they can focus their energy on the hard work of improving lives.[144]

For as Do No Harm member Wes Ogilvie, a paramedic and attorney in Austin, Texas, asks, "Does a class on implicit bias best serve the patients I take care of? If I take that class versus one on patient care documentation, which course offers more benefit to my patients, myself, or the organization I'm with?"

To ask that question is to answer it.

The snipe hunt for implicit bias blinds us to the very real problems that beset healthcare for many minority persons. Pointing this out is a surefire way of earning time in the pillory, as I learned when I somewhat rashly tweeted on the subject. (I have since become more careful about tweets; one flippant crack—however truthful—calls forth the crazies and the cancelers.)

The Michigan course was put together by Do No Harm's Laura Morgan, a terrific nurse who was fired from her job with Baylor Scott & White Health, a Dallas-based healthcare system, because she would not submit to implicit bias haranguing.

Laura's case is poignant and frightening. Offended by the demand that she take a newly mandatory course called "Overcoming Unconscious Bias," she asked for a waiver. Laura explained, "After 39 years of providing equal care to all my patients without regard to their race, I objected to a mandatory course grounded in the idea that I'm racist because I'm white."

For upholding her principles, Laura was fired. "I went from a six-figure job to zero income," she says. "The day I was fired I sold my car to make sure I'd have enough money to live on. When I tried to find a

---

144 Stanley Goldfarb, "How We've Taken the Bias Out of 'Implicit Bias Training,'" *Wall Street Journal*, April 26, 2024.

new healthcare job, no one would hire me. No doubt if they contacted my old employer, they were told why I was let go."

Laura discovered that hers was not an isolated case. And deep blue states like Massachusetts and Maryland aren't the only ones to impose implicit bias training on healthcare professionals. For instance, the Kentucky Board of Nursing forces all registered nurses to submit to implicit bias education. The Kentucky Nurses Association's course is the one that teaches that "implicit bias kills" and that a nurse's actions may contribute to "modern-day lynchings in the workplace."

Meekly assenting to these absurdities and outright lies is the price a Kentucky nurse pays for keeping his or her job. (The indoctrination and pressure to conform on nurses is even stronger than for doctors. Nurses aren't quite as independent as doctors; they tend to be working under the guidance of physicians. Their organizations are often woke to the nth degree.)

Laura Morgan saw a grim future: "I fear every healthcare professional will soon be forced to make the same awful decision I did: Falsely admit to being racist or abandon the medical field."[145]

Laura refused to roll over. Instead, she joined Do No Harm as our program manager and designed the two-hour online Michigan course, whose popularity has exceeded our expectations. Over two thousand Michigan health professionals have taken the course—and we've only just begun.

We've dotted all the bureaucratic i's and crossed the t's, meeting the state of Michigan's criteria for those offering an implicit bias course. If the DEI fanatics within state government try to decertify us we will sue for viewpoint discrimination. And as I write, Do No Harm is looking into expanding this to other states.

For those lacking, at least at present, the Michigan option, Do No Harm has compiled a handy list of actions you can take if your medical

---

[145] Laura L. Morgan, "'Implicit Bias' Training Cost Me My Nursing Job," *Wall Street Journal*, September 30, 2022.

school, state licensing board, or healthcare employer pushes you to take implicit bias training or testing.

These include:

1—Ask if the training is mandatory, and if so, why. This allows you to avoid it if it's not required.

2—Ask if you can receive an alternative accommodation, such as writing an essay on equality under the law or the danger of "anti-racist" discrimination. This allows you to push back on the faulty logic that underlies implicit bias.

3—Share materials on how implicit bias testing has been discredited. You can find a trove of resources at the Do No Harm website that will arm you with arguments about why this ideologically driven agenda shouldn't be forced on you and your fellow medical professionals and employees. You might say to those ordering you to submit to this propaganda:

Why are medical professionals like me being pushed to take a test that is widely recognized as faulty? It would be far better to avoid this test altogether—and for that matter, to avoid implicitly or explicitly telling me and my peers that we're biased because of our skin color. That reeks of discrimination in and of itself and is wholly inappropriate for healthcare.

I hope you make the right call and abandon the Implicit Association Test. Thanks for looking into this urgent and important matter.

4—Decline to attend an in-person training or complete an online training. Even if the training is required, you should share your concerns with your supervisors.

5—Take careful notes and obtain copies of the training materials. If you are forced to participate, you can share what happened after the fact with Do No Harm to help prevent it from happening again.

6—Ask direct questions that highlight the divisive and discriminatory nature of implicit bias training. That includes asking why "anti-racism" requires you to discriminate on the basis of race, which hotline or agency you should call to report such discrimination, and what evidence exists that proves you are inherently biased or racist. There are many pointed questions you can ask in these trainings:

— *The main proponent of "anti-racism," Ibram X. Kendi, has explicitly said that racial discrimination is acceptable. Here is his quote: "The only remedy to past discrimination is present discrimination. The only remedy to present discrimination is future discrimination." What discriminatory actions are you asking me to take in my day-to-day work as a healthcare professional?*

— *How does "anti-racist" discrimination square with our duty to provide equal care to all patients, regardless of skin color? Please help me understand which forms of discrimination are acceptable, and which are not, according to our employee handbook and human resources department.*

— *The concept of implicit bias is directly tied to the "Implicit Association Test." Yet diverse psychologists from across the political spectrum have thoroughly discredited the test. Even its own creators have said it can't actually be used to predict individuals' behavior. Given these facts, why are we being requested or forced to take this test?*

— *The concept of implicit bias is directly tied to the principles of "anti-racism," which require some groups of people to discriminate against other groups based solely on skin color. For years, healthcare providers have been trained to treat patients ethically*

and fairly with no mention of "anti-racism." Given these facts,
why are we being requested or forced to take this course?

7—Alert your state and federal lawmakers. Tell them what's happening and why it's dangerous, so they can investigate and shine a light on the inappropriate and dangerous woke agenda.

The bottom line is that you *can* push back on implicit bias training. Ideological indoctrination has no place in healthcare—and it's up to us to reteach the medical world this fundamental and essential truth.

It seems incredible that the American healthcare system would expel skilled and dedicated practitioners for political reasons, but Laura Morgan is far from the only health professional to have been fired for objecting to implicit bias training.

Brad McDowell was a registered nurse and assistant clinical manager in the emergency room at Meritus Medical Center in Hagerstown, Maryland. "Since I oversaw nurses, my highest priority after providing the best care to patients was protecting my team," says Brad. And that's what got him in trouble.

Maryland mandates implicit bias training for medical professionals. Its professed goal is to reduce the maternal mortality gap between black and non-black women.

Brad recalls:

> I took the first session of the course in July 2023. I was bombarded with evidence-free claims that implicit bias has caused a crisis of maternal mortality in black women. The course ignored the complex factors that contribute to higher black maternal mortality, including comorbidities, while defining any death from any cause after a year of giving birth as maternal mortality—a logical stretch.

Overall, the course implied that white nurses like me are killing black mothers. I was supposed to internalize this message and somehow apply it to the management of my team.

Several months later, Brad received a batch of materials for the next DEI brainwashing session, this one for hospital leaders like Brad. These included the statement that the United States is built on "an ideology of White supremacy that justifies policies, practices and structures which result in social arrangements of subordination for groups of color through power and White privilege."

Refusing to subject his nurses to this libelous bilge, Brad boycotted the session. He also refused to attend the next implicit bias training session. He was punished for neither action—he was a valuable member of the emergency room health team, after all—but when Brad criticized implicit bias on his Facebook page, civilly and without mentioning his employer, he was placed on administrative leave and then fired.

Brad, who I am proud to say is a member of Do No Harm, described his plight in the *Wall Street Journal*:

> I'm 47. I have many good years left in the workforce. I want to keep doing what I have always done, which is to provide the highest level of care to patients of every race, ethnicity and background. I also want to keep leading diverse teams, helping them become better nurses regardless of what they look like or whom they treat.
>
> In the meeting where I was fired, a Meritus representative repeatedly said I had waded into 'a touchy subject.' That's exactly my point. DEI is inherently divisive and discriminatory to boot. No hospital or medical provider

should touch something so touchy, much less fire someone for daring to question it.[146]

Clete Weigel, a nurse in Kent, Ohio, has also paid the price for
bravely dissenting from the party line.

In 2023, the diversity director at Summa Health, Clete's employer,
announced that the hospital would implement implicit bias training
"to reduce health disparities." The diversity director invited a response
on her blog, so Clete responded with statistical and observational data
about the reality of health disparities. He also challenged the efficacy of
implicit bias training.

His blog post was never seen by the workforce. Instead, he was sum-
moned to a meeting and informed of his punishment: he would have
to undergo not one but *two* implicit bias trainings! (Interesting, isn't it,
that those administering it regard additional implicit bias training as a
punishment?)

After thirty-seven years of service as an award-winning nurse, Clete
Weigel resigned. He told Do No Harm:

> Hospital leaders have chosen to make operational deci-
> sions based upon ideology. Logic and arguments do not
> matter; the ideology does. Everything becomes second-
> ary when ideology rules. That includes evidence-based
> medicine, valuing employees, science, discernment, the
> exchange of ideas, and yes, common-sense.
>
> Medicine will not be served by this ideology. Patients
> will be harmed by a worldview that prefers narratives
> over science and identity groups over individuals. In the
> end, individual care will suffer as implicit bias training

---

146 Brad McDowell, "DEI Got Me Sacked From My Nursing Job," *Wall Street Journal*,
March 15, 2024.

increases suspicion, discourse devolves, and patients are neglected.

This is not an abstract matter. Lives—and livelihoods—are at stake.

Dr. Jared Ross, an emergency physician, assistant professor at the University of Missouri, and member of Do No Harm, currently faces an end to his livelihood unless he confesses what he believes to be a falsehood. Dr. Ross must sign a code in which he pledges to "mitigate both implicit or explicit biases based on race, gender, age, sexual orientation, disability, national origin, or religion providing patient care." If he refuses to do so when his certification is up for renewal by the American Board of Emergency Medicine in 2029, he will lose his license—and his community will lose a good doctor, just because he resists compelled speech.

Dr. Ross is a man of courage and principle. With respect to this modern version of a 1950s loyalty oath, he says:

> I can't mitigate something that I don't believe exists in the first place. But if you start challenging things like implicit bias, you are putting your livelihood at risk. There are plenty of things we can debate as emergency physicians—we can have an academic discussion about the best antibiotics to treat an open fracture, or what medication should be first line for atrial fibrillation with rapid ventricular response. But DEI is not open for discussion.

Jared knows the risks of not signing the code. Losing his certification would make it hard, if not impossible, to work in any sort of hospital or medical establishment, even as an outside consultant. He's still not going to sign it.

"They are looking for me to engage in racism and sexism in the name of equity. But equity and equality are inherently incompatible," he says. "I won't do it. It's dangerous."

Does anyone but the most foaming-at-the-mouth fanatic want to argue that American healthcare is better off without Laura Morgan, Brad McDowell, Clete Weigel, and Jared Ross?

- - - - - -

Do black people need black doctors? No, black people, like people of all races, need competent doctors, no matter the race.

It is a measure of the topsy-turviness of DEI-driven discourse that this is a controversial statement.

Racial concordance, or lack thereof, has been pushed as one reason for disparities in health outcomes between blacks and other racial groups.

This is treated as gospel truth by the corporate media. *CBS Evening News*, for example, kicked off a report with the wholly unsupported assertion that "More diversity among cardiologists would save lives." It relayed without a trace of skepticism the statement of Dr. Michelle Albert, president of the American Heart Association, that "structural racism and the fact that persons of color have been systematically excluded from being part of the process that enables you to become a doctor in the first place" are the reasons that the percentage of black cardiologists (3 percent) is well below the percentage of black Americans (13 percent) in the general population.[147]

CNN, meanwhile, says that the fact that 5.7 percent of American doctors are black "harms public health"—or so "experts warn." (When a journalist quotes an "expert" it is always, without fail, to confirm the opinion of the journalist.) According to the Associated Press, "experts" also say "diversity is especially needed within specialty medicine."[148]

---

[147] Adriana Diaz, "Black cardiologists are rare, but vital for Black patients," CBS Evening News, February 16, 2023; Claretta Bellamy, "Black people have the highest rates of death from heart disease. Could more Black cardiologists help?" NBC News, February 19, 2024.

[148] Kat Stafford, "Patients need doctors who look like them. Can medicine diversify without affirmative action?" Associated Press, September 10, 2023.

The incommensurate percentage of black doctors is said to be a legacy of American medicine's "deep-rooted history of racism," as evidenced by the minuscule proportion (1.3 percent) of black physicians in 1900 and 1940 (2.8 percent). (Virtually all of these early pioneer black physicians were male.)[149]

A factoid bruited about by some DEI advocates has it that the odds of a black patient seeing a black doctor are about forty times greater than those of a black patient seeing a white doctor. One natural reaction to this information would be, "Who cares? What does it matter?" Dr. William McDade, who bears the ominous title of chief diversity and inclusion officer at the American Council for Graduate Medical Education, says he cares and it matters because "people prefer physicians of their own race and ethnicity, speaking in their own primary language."[150]

Is the implication here that black and white Americans speak different languages? Except in the case of people recently immigrated, this is awfully unlikely.

So in one of our first projects, Do No Harm examined the evidence for the proposition that patients achieve better outcomes when treated by doctors of the same race—and we found it thin, if not nonexistent. Critical race theory demands of its adherents the subordination of facts to theory. Consider: there are now dozens of studies of whether black patients and black doctors communicate better than when the dyad consists of a white physician and a black patient.

In all, there have been five systematic reviews of these racial concordance studies. The most recent, which appeared in the journal *Health Communication*, surveyed thirty-three such studies and concluded, "Race/ethnicity concordance with their physician does not appear to

149 Jacqueline Howard, "Only 5.75% of US doctors are Black, and experts warn the shortage harms public health," CNN Health, February 21, 2023; Dan P. Ly, "Historical Trends in the Representativeness and Incomes of Black Physicians, 1900-2018," *Journal of General Internal Medicine* 37, no. 5 (April 2022): 1310–1312.

150 Len Strazewski, "Why physician diversity matters, and how GME programs can boost it," AMA, July 20, 2021.

influence the quality of communication for most patients from minoritized groups."[151]

Three of the four earlier systematic studies reached much the same conclusion. Salimah H. Meghani et al., writing in *Ethnicity & Health*, discerned "no clear patterns" in the relationship between racial concordance and health outcomes in the twenty-seven studies they examined.[152] Similarly, Sonia V. Otte and her fellow researchers, writing in the *Journal of Patient Experience*, explained that most of the fourteen racial concordance studies under review "resulted in no significant association between patient–provider racial concordance and improved patient outcomes. Racially concordant care did not affect factors such as quality of surgical care, hospitalist performance, patient trust, and quality of care outcomes (i.e., trust, satisfaction, and decision-making propensity)."[153] And in an extensive examination of studies of surgical patient experiences published in the journal *Surgery*, Cindy Zhao et al. reported "no effect of race concordance on the quality of care."[154]

The outlier in the quintet of systematic studies appeared in 2018 in the *Journal of Racial and Ethnic Health Disparities*. Affirming the positive effect of racial concordance, this paper omitted (for unclear reasons) studies that should have qualified for inclusion and was hampered by curious and inconsistent categorizations.[155]

---

[151] Ann Neville Miller et al., "The Relationship of Race/Ethnicity Concordance to Physician-Patient Communication: A Mixed-Methods Systematic Review," *Health Communication* 39, no. 8 (2024): 1543–1557.

[152] Salimah H. Meghani et al., "Patient–provider race-concordance: does it matter in improving minority patients' health outcomes?" *Ethnicity & Health* 14, no. 1 (January 2009): 107–130.

[153] Sonia V. Otte, "Improved Patient Experience and Outcomes: Is Patient–Provider Concordance the Key?" *Journal of Patient Experience* (2022): 9.

[154] Cindy Zhao et al., "Race, gender, and language concordance in the care of surgical patients: A systematic review," *Surgery* 166, no. 5 (November 2019): 785–792.

[155] Megan Johnson Shen et al., "The Effects of Race and Racial Concordance on Patient-Physician Communication: A Systematic Review of the Literature," *Journal of Racial and Ethnic Health Disparities* 5, no. 1 (February 2018): 117–140.

This last-named study seems to cherry-pick. (DEI partisans are cherry-pickers par excellence.)[156] Yet in the face of overwhelming evidence, DEI bureaucrats still claim that more black physicians are required in order to improve health outcomes. Do we really want white patients entering healthcare institutions and demanding that they only see white physicians? I witnessed bigoted patients making such demands during my days as a clinician. When patients made such demands at our hospital, we told them to seek another hospital.

Another consequence of this model is the conclusion that black patients don't seek the best medical care and are more interested in the race of their healthcare providers. How demeaning to black patients!

Racial concordance lumps people of vastly different backgrounds and experiences into one undifferentiated mass called "black." A highly educated doctor from an upper-class Nigerian family will have very little in common with a poor black mother from inner-city Oakland. They may get along fine, but there is certainly the potential for a culture clash, or at least a cultural misalignment. And the idea that a Jewish doctor will necessarily work in perfect harmony with a Jewish patient is nonsense—as I can testify from firsthand experience.

These easy alliances on the basis of race or religion are just not how the world works. As Do No Harm member Rodney Long Jr., an Ohio mental health therapist, observes, "Everybody has *somebody* they can look to and rely on for guidance and support. The problem is that we start saying things like, 'well, you're not black, so you don't understand.' Or, 'You didn't grow up poor, so you don't understand.' Let me tell you, none of the people who helped me out the most were from where I was from. The most influential people in my life were people who were not like me."

Those who believe in racial concordance—and impose this belief on medical schools and, ultimately, patients—point to one flawed study to buttress their opinion. This pivotal study is used to promote the idea

---

[156] Kingsbury and Greene, "The Return of Segregation."

that patients should generally or even exclusively see physicians of the same race, which is tantamount to segregation.

The study that forms the flimsy foundation of the racial concordance industry has so many flaws—and they go so manifestly unreported by DEI advocates—that it is worth examining in some detail.[157]

"Does Diversity Matter? Experimental Evidence from Oakland," the medical study heard 'round the world, was published first in June 2018 and then in a revised version in the December 2019 issue of the respected *American Economic Review*.[158] Its three authors posited that black physicians treat black patients better than white or Asian physicians do, all else being equal. Its central claim has been used to justify the aggressive push for racial diversity in medical schools and residency and training programs.

The study's findings are startling. The authors state that racially matching physicians and patients "could lead to a 19 percent reduction in the black-white male cardiovascular mortality gap and an 8 percent decline in the black-white male life expectancy gap." The healthcare community responded to this shocking conclusion with hasty and ill-advised action. For instance, despite an internal survey finding fierce opposition from physicians and consumers, UnitedHealth Group, the largest health insurance company in America by revenue, is in the process of publicly collecting and disseminating the race of physicians to incentivize patients to choose a healthcare provider of the same race.

But the Oakland study can't prove what it wants to prove, namely that black patients should seek out black doctors for better health outcomes.

Despite its flaws, the study holds sway, and for a good reason. Medical journals are almost entirely hostile to arguments that push back

---

[157] Thanks to Alexander Raikin, Senior Fellow at Do No Harm, with whom I collaborated on "Re-Segregating Healthcare: Finding the Flaws in a Famous—and Dangerous—Study," Do No Harm, August 26, 2022.

[158] Marcella Alsan, Owen Garrick, and Grant Graziani, "Does Diversity Matter for Health? Experimental Evidence from Oakland," *American Economic Review* 109, no. 12 (December 2019): 4071–4111.

on the paradigms of anti-racism and DEI, which is the foundation of the Oakland study. Indeed, one article that found a weakness in the study was retracted. Its author, Norman Wang, was "canceled" by the cardiology community, in part over his critique of the Oakland study. Yet the major flaws in the design and interpretation of the Oakland study call into question its conclusion, which rejects the long-standing scientific consensus that a physician's race has no relevant impact on health outcomes.

Institutionally segregating physicians by race damages the trust between physicians and patients. This poorly designed and executed study wrongly tells black patients that non-black physicians are less able to treat their illnesses—even when such a physician might be the most qualified or appropriate one for the situation. For black physicians, this study implies that even when they perform better than non-black doctors, it is not because of the quality of their medical expertise, but rather because their work is, to a significant degree, skin-deep. The Oakland study gives an imprimatur to medical institutions as they inch closer to the slippery slope of race-based medicine. To medical researchers, it shows that scientific claims can be exaggerated beyond their logical premises in the pursuit of a cause they deem worthy. And to white patients, it raises the ugly possibility that they should seek out white doctors to achieve optimum health outcomes.

The Oakland study was designed to test prospectively whether black patients would accept preventative recommendations at higher rates if they were made by a black physician. Black men were recruited from mostly black barbershops in Oakland, California, with a small financial incentive to come to a medical clinic for a preventative check-up. When they arrived, they were shown a computer tablet with a male doctor's name and photo (black or white) and were told to select which preventative service they would be willing to accept. They could pick either an invasive procedure like cholesterol or diabetes testing (requiring a blood draw) and a flu shot, or some non-invasive tests like measuring blood pressure or body mass index (BMI).

The patients subsequently met their assigned physician, either black or white. The physician was instructed to try to convince each patient to accept as many preventative services as possible. The Oakland researchers compared the difference in willingness of the patients to engage in the preventative services before and after they met with their assigned doctors. The key outcome was whether the patients who saw a black doctor were more willing to undergo the preventative tests than those who saw a white doctor.

The Oakland study reported that black patients chose more preventative services, especially those that were more invasive, from black physicians than from white physicians. The authors went on to speculate that the increased willingness to undergo preventative services, if applied to the entire national cohort of black men, would produce dramatic improvements in morbidity and mortality of black Americans.

Alas, the Oakland study is riddled with manifold flaws. First off, it has no control group.

While it is commendable that the authors managed to recruit over 1,300 black men from twenty black barbershops and two flea markets, the study's design makes it impossible to distinguish the effect of unobserved covariates like the relative effectiveness of the individual black versus non-black physicians in persuading patients. A control group consisting of white patients experiencing the same test conditions is necessary to assess whether the black doctors were more effective because they were black, or because they were better communicators.

The authors realized this problem, but they did so too late to solve it. Instead, they post-facto tried to produce a small study within a study and use the twelve non-black patients who were recruited incidentally as a pseudo-control group. However, there is a fundamental problem: These non-black men likely had unobservable and observable characteristics that differ from the sample of black men. They were not recruited to match the experimental group in important characteristics like age and underlying health status.

To prove that the race of the physician matters, it is necessary to prove that other factors don't—the most obvious being that a physician is better at his or her job due to skills instead of skin color. Consequently, a control group of non-black patients is crucial, as it would help determine whether some doctors were simply more persuasive across all race groups.

A second flaw is that the samples were unrepresentative.

Surprisingly, the patients who chose to participate in this experiment were apparently healthier than the average black person in America. This doesn't make sense for several reasons. The patients who came to the clinic were 60 percent more likely to be uninsured and 340 percent more likely to be unemployed than the average black person in America. Yet their blood pressure, BMI, cholesterol levels, and blood glucose values were, on average, lower than the typical black man in America.

The obvious reason for this disparity is self-selection bias. It seems likely that patients selected the screening tests that they believed they would pass, perhaps either for their own self-image or because they believed that good results would secure the financial incentive. Alternatively, the unhealthiest participants were more likely to have chosen not to participate in the study. Someone who was overweight might have opted for a blood pressure measurement (which he might or might not pass) versus a BMI measurement, which he knows would show that he is overweight.

Most damningly, the doctors involved in the study were not representative of the wider physician population. Only eight non-black doctors and six black doctors were used. The authors use percentages to imply a far larger sample, noting in one case that 67 percent of black doctors in the study were internal medicine doctors—but that simply means that four out of six doctors were internists. To state the obvious, such a non-representative sample of doctors is not generalizable to the medical field writ large.

Furthermore, the authors take unproven logical leaps. They rely on a dubious and unproven projection of the value of and subjects' long-term adherence to preventative healthcare services. They argue that "part of the mortality disparity [between non-Blacks and Blacks] is related to underutilized preventative healthcare services" and these preventative services can be represented by five one-time tests (flu vaccine, blood pressure measurement, BMI measurement, cholesterol testing, and diabetes testing). Based on this, the researchers extrapolate huge increases in black life expectancy from physician-patient racial concordance.

This is highly doubtful. Preventative screening is only effective if used in a patient who has a high likelihood of being at risk for a particular clinical condition and who is committed to following any recommended treatments. A healthy, young, non-obese man does not need to be screened for diabetes; similarly, someone who had a normal cholesterol level six months ago would not necessarily need another test.

More importantly, not only is the one-time use of these five tests not necessarily part of proper preventative services, but it does not define a well-rounded set of preventative services. Primary interventions, like the tests administered, are only a minor component of such services. They need to be combined with lifestyle changes and, possibly, compliance with a consistent medication regime to be effective. All the health outcomes of the procedures performed in this experiment, apart from the flu shot, rely on modifying what patients do in the future: alter their activity level, reduce their weight, and possibly employ antihypertensive medication. Yet there was no attempt to record the impact of these one-time interventions with a follow-up survey.

Why would black Americans not use preventative medical care? The Oakland researchers suggest that current African American mistrust of medical care is caused by racist historical events, notably the Tuskegee syphilis experiments. (The authors say that a subject's rejection of a flu shot because he feared "being experimented on" was "a possible reference to the syphilis experiment in Tuskegee." But his suspicion could have reflected contemporary anti-vaccine dialogue.) To test this claim that American blacks are most influenced by the history of events like the Tuskegee experiments, one can compare the health and economic status of blacks in the United States with a similar country without an extended history of slavery and segregation, such as Canada. This involves comparing the health of black immigrants to Canada and the United States. (Canada accepts a relatively more highly skilled group of immigrants, so it is necessary to make statistical adjustments for education and other covariates.) The finding of one such promising study is that the rates of social and economic integration "are virtually identical" in almost all supposed social determinants of health, ranging from social equality to income.[159] Consequently, it seems unlikely that the mistrust black Americans have derives from past historical events. Instead, any mistrust would have to be based on current phenomena, and the researchers did not attempt to make or support this argument.

The most uncomfortable problem presented by the study is this: How does the mechanism of black doctors interacting with black patients increase health outcomes? The authors try their hardest to avoid claiming that either the patients or the doctors are racist (in academese, they call it "taste-based discrimination"). Patients, for instance, had no preference for doctors with their own racial background before they met their assigned doctor; all doctors were rated highly at the end of the study. But why is it then that black patients would trust black doctors more than non-black doctors, if both sets of doctors were regarded as trustworthy? The proposed mechanism of easier communication presupposes the racial essentialism that a black man must have something in common with another black man solely because of his race. If the

---

[159] Jeffery G. Reitz, "Multiculturalism Policies and Popular Multiculturalism in the Development of Canadian Immigration," September 2013, https://www.yumpu.com/en/document/view/51633638/, accessed August 1, 2022.

assertions for the Oakland paper are true, then it seems that "taste-based discrimination" is the guiding phenomenon for health outcomes—which the researchers deny.

Despite these disabling flaws, the Oakland study rapidly gained canonical stature. One of its authors, Marcella Alsan, received a MacArthur Foundation "genius" grant after its publication. Her jaw-droppingly baseless conclusion that racial concordance would lower cardiovascular deaths among black men by 19 percent boggles the mind, but I guess that passes for genius in the 2020s.

Common sense implies that the academic medical community would not merely praise a paper but would offer an evenhanded approach. Without skepticism, the scientific method is impossible: the pursuit of truth requires well-founded criticism to probe the weaknesses and strengths of any argument, even more if we believe the claim in question. If something sounds true, there must be evidence that it is true. Yet the Oakland study has been all but unchallenged, even as its unproven assumptions and faulty design have formed the foundation of subsequent medical research.

Only Norman Wang's study discussed potential problems with the Oakland study. Wang stated:

> The results have little external validity as the study only involved 14 physicians (8 non-Black and 6 Black). Moreover, mortality estimates were extrapolated from single patient-physician encounters using methods so unscientific that the investigators themselves described them as "back-of-the-envelope calculation."[160]

But here, too, the story takes a twist. Norman Wang's paper was retracted almost six months after the American Heart Association published

---

[160] Norman Wang, "Diversity, Inclusion, and Equity: Evolution of Race and Ethnicity Considerations for the Cardiology Workforce in the United States of America From 1969 to 2019," *Journal of the American Heart Association* 9, no. 7 (2020).

it. The AHA said the article "contains many misconceptions and misquotes and that together those inaccuracies, misstatements, and selective misreading of source materials void the paper of its scientific validity."[161]

Wang rejects this characterization. He believes that his essay was retracted because he opposes affirmative action in cardiology programs, which led to him being fired from his leadership positions and disciplined by his academic institution. It has become academic suicide to claim, as Wang does, that "all who aspire to a profession in medicine and cardiology must be assessed as individuals on the basis of their personal merits, not their racial and ethnic identities." Fittingly, this brouhaha occurred in 2020, when wokeness was at an apex.

My suspicion is that most who use the Oakland study to promote racial concordance have never actually read it. Perhaps they've perused the abstract and conclusion, at most. Those are the easy parts of the study to read; they don't require analyzing data. They require no independent judgment at all.

What we have here is confirmation bias. The paper's conclusions support the ideological prejudices of DEI advocates and affirm their worldview. There is no search for truth, just a search for justification.

Dramatic claims require dramatic evidence to be credible. The evidence presented by the Oakland study does not support its conclusions.

Yes, the Oakland study produced an interesting finding. It suggests something—namely, that another study be done, a wider study with a different population to see if you get the same results with a different set of doctors. That's the next step. The next step is *not* to change the entire healthcare system because of this study.

In sum, the Oakland study is not a landmark paper that proves the United States must train more black physicians to achieve better health outcomes for black patients, much less push patients to rely

---

[161] "Retraction to: Diversity, Inclusion, and Equity: Evolution of Race and Ethnicity Considerations for the Cardiology Workforce in the United States of America From 1969 to 2019," *Journal of the American Heart Association* 9, no. 20 (2020).

primarily or solely on physicians of their own race or gender. Rather, it is an unproven and unpersuasive effort to convince policymakers of a dubious plan to make racial concordance a reality in American healthcare—which in essence means a return to racial segregation of medical care. The Oakland study should have been challenged by an army of researchers: people who typically demand rigor in design and interpretation before they accept studies as definitive. Instead, it was treated with broad and unthinking acceptance. The mounting campaign for a twenty-first-century segregation of healthcare is dangerous and baseless. The Oakland study does not change that fact.

Ultimately, black patients want the best doctors and the best medical care more than they desire doctors that are racially concordant. Competence, not color, is what matters.

The high price exacted by race-obsessed medicine was visible in tragic outline at the Martin Luther King Jr./Drew Medical Center near Watts, which was founded in 1972 near the site of the famous 1965 Los Angeles race riots.

A team of *Los Angeles Times* reporters won a Pulitzer Prize for its investigation into what had become known as "Killer King." The hospital, which had been the object of frequent civil rights complaints that it discriminated in hiring and promotion against non-minority doctors, had to close in 2007, a victim of almost mind-numbing incompetence.

In 2004, the *Los Angeles Times* summarized Killer King's crimes against its patients:

— "Errors and neglect by King/Drew's staff have repeatedly injured or killed patients over more than a decade, a pattern that remains largely unscrutinized and unchecked. Some lapses were never reported to authorities—or even to the victims or their families. And some people learned of the severity of the failings only by suing or, in several instances, from *Times* reporters who sought them out to learn about their care."

— "Although King/Drew opened in 1972 with the promise that it would be 'the very best hospital in America,' it is now, by various measures, one of the very worst. It pays out more per patient for medical malpractice than any of the state's 17 other public hospitals or the six University of California medical centers."

— "Entire departments are riddled with incompetence, internal strife and, in some cases, criminality. Employees have pilfered and sometimes sold the hospital's drugs; chronic absenteeism is rampant; assaults between hospital workers are not uncommon. Despite King/Drew's repeated promises to regulators, the problems have gone unfixed for years."

— "The hospital's failings do not stem from a lack of money, as its supporters long have contended. King/Drew spends more per patient than any of the three other general hospitals run by Los Angeles County. Millions of dollars go to unusual workers' compensation claims and abnormally high salaries for ranking doctors."

— "The hospital's governing body, the county Board of Supervisors, has been told repeatedly—often in writing—of needless deaths and injuries at King/Drew. Recently the supervisors have made some aggressive moves aimed at fixing the hospital. But for years, the board shied away from decisive action in the face of community anger and accusations of racism."[162]

Subordination of competence to DEI brings about atrocities like Killer King.

---

[162] Tracy Weber, Charles Ornstein, and Mitchell Landsberg, "Deadly errors and politics betray a hospital's promise," *Los Angeles Times*, December 5, 2004.

- - - - - -

Being a membership organization offers Do No Harm an effective way to challenge unconstitutional DEI programs in instances where our members have legal standing.

We see discrimination and we sue. The heroic labors of Kristina Rasmussen often enable us to find the plaintiffs in these suits. While working at the Illinois Policy Institute, Kristina found Mark Janus, the Illinois social worker who lent his name to *Janus v. AFSCME* (2018), a landmark workers' rights case decided by the US Supreme Court. Do No Harm's seventeen thousand members offer a rich potential plaintiff pool, and they are a tremendous resource when we put out a call for, say, an ob-gyn in California.

Consovoy McCarthy, one of the leading conservatively inclined civil rights law firms in the country, represented us in one of our first big lawsuits.

The issue concerned Medicare. In late 2021, the Biden Administration's Department of Health and Human Services posted updates to Medicare's Merit-based Incentive Payment System that directed Medicare to provide an incremental payment under its quality improvement program to physicians who had established an anti-discrimination, anti-racism protocol in their practice. The intent of the rule-makers was to encourage doctors "to acknowledge systemic racism as a root cause for differences in health outcomes between socially-defined racial groups."[163]

The details were vague, but the idea was that a physician would be rewarded for treating patients differently depending on their race. It could be something as innocuous or even meritorious as having a translator in your practice, or it might go all the way to favoring patients on the basis of the color of their skin. In return for acting on racist principles, doctors would be reimbursed for their services at a higher rate.

---

[163] Alec Schemmel, "HHS allows doctors implementing 'anti-racism plan' to charge more for services," Fox News, December 18, 2021, https://fox11online.com/.

Many doctors were outraged by this, and as they had standing we sued the federal government on their behalf. The wheels of justice can grind slowly; Do No Harm's case, *Colville v. Becerra*, which takes its name from plaintiff Dr. Amber Colville, a Mississippi physician, is still working its way through the courts.

Coincidentally, I recently found myself on a plane sitting next to Lee Fleisher. Lee, who had been a colleague at Penn, later went to work as the chief medical officer and director of the Centers for Medicare and Medicaid Services Center for Clinical Standards and Quality.

"Hi, Lee," I chirped, glad to see an old Penn hand. "Do you remember me?"

"Do I remember you?" he replied. "You sued me!"

Oops—Lee's bailiwick included the Merit-based Incentive Payment System.

After the initial awkwardness we had a pleasant conversation.

The target of our second lawsuit was *Health Affairs*, a prominent journal of healthcare policy.

Like much of the clerisy, the editors of *Health Affairs* went off the rails in the summer of Black Lives Matter. They beat their breasts, they donned the hairshirt, they announced that minority voices must be heard. The DEI playbook was in full flower. Soon enough they came out with a Health Equity Fellowship for Trainees which was open only to applicants who "identify as American Indian/Alaskan Native, African American/Black, Asian American, Native Hawaiian and other Pacific Islander, and Hispanic/Latino."[164]

This was a plum fellowship with a nice stipend attached, offering those chosen the opportunity to learn the workings of medical journals from the inside. But whites need not apply. For all its self-serving talk of anti-racism and inclusion, *Health Affairs* was engaging in illegal and immoral racial discrimination.

---

[164] Do No Harm, "*Health Affairs* Drops Racial Fellowship Requirements Following Do No Harm Lawsuit," press release, January 22, 2024.

Since *Health Affairs'* publishing organization, Project HOPE, accepts federal funding, it is subject to the ban on racial discrimination under the federal Civil Rights Act, which states: "No person in the United States shall, on the ground of race, color, or national origin, be excluded from participation in, be denied the benefits of, or be subjected to discrimination under any program or activity receiving Federal financial assistance."

As if that weren't enough law-breaking, *Health Affairs* and Project HOPE were also running afoul of the Affordable Care Act, and *Health Affairs* was violating DC law, which prohibits racial discrimination in training programs.

I was sitting in a pub in Ireland when I received an email from the editor of *Health Affairs* asking me for evidence that his journal had said what we said they had said. I texted our research director, who texted back, and I forwarded the evidence. The editor himself had proposed the discriminatory practices in a forgotten editorial!

The editors of *Health Affairs*, who could read the writing on the wall, eliminated the unlawful requirement, and as a result Do No Harm voluntarily dismissed our lawsuit without prejudice.

Do No Harm bought an ad in the August 2022 number of *Health Affairs* asking why the journal was discriminating against unfavored races. We told its readers, "Here's your chance to resist this destructive trend—and to protect healthcare for doctors and patients."

This gave the *Health Affairs* editor a chance to exercise his sanctimony muscle, taking our money while condemning Do No Harm and everything he believed we stood for. It was high dudgeon in its lowest form.

Editor Alan Weil delivered a less than gripping account of the ethical conundrum he faced in deciding whether to accept a paid advertisement from an organization with which he disagreed. For editors operating from a pro–free speech, let-a-thousand-flowers-bloom perspective—which is disappearing in intolerantly woke America—this is an easy choice. Take the money and let those with whom you disagree have their say.

But Weil apparently tossed and turned and spent many a sleepless night pondering this choice. Finally, he consented to take our money, but "did so with mixed feelings after considerable deliberation." You see, in his view we rejected "the existence of, and the harms associated with, racism."

This is flatly untrue. Racism in America, though obviously less virulent today than in, say, the Deep South of the 1950s, is unfortunately still with us, and we categorically reject any government policies based in or promoting racism or racial favoritism.

Weil went on to wail, "It was obvious to us that if we declined the ad, we too would be criticized for our decision. The victimization narrative, which they promote so heavily on their website, would have one more entry. And the story would be theirs to tell."[165]

Note that a commitment to the free exchange of ideas was not enough to motivate acceptance of the ad.

— — — — — —

One of our potentially most consequential lawsuits is against Pfizer, which followed the corporate crowd in going full-on woke. Pfizer announced a whites-and-Asians-need-not-apply fellowship through which the pharmaceutical giant would fund master's degrees for these fellows and then presumably bring them into the company.

This was a clear, even blatant violation of Title VI of the Civil Rights Act of 1964, which prohibits discrimination on the basis of race, color, and national origin in programs and activities receiving federal financial assistance. A private company like Pfizer is fair game for a suit if it accepts funds from the federal government. If there were a threshold,

---

[165] Alan Weil, "Minimizing Harm: Why We Published An Ad We Found Objectionable," *Health Affairs*, August 4, 2022.

Pfizer, as a charter member of Big Pharma, would easily exceed it, but in fact there is no minimum or percentage requirement. Take the king's shilling, become the king's man, as the old saying goes.

As it happens, a young Do No Harm member of one of the proscribed racial groups wished to apply for the Pfizer fellowship. Alas, he or she had the wrong genes. So Do No Harm leapt into action, suing on this person's behalf, keeping his or her identity anonymous.

To show how seriously Pfizer took the suit, it bought the services of Loretta Lynch, who had served as US attorney general under President Barack Obama. The district court dismissed our case on the grounds that Do No Harm lacked standing. We appealed to the US Court of Appeals for the Second Circuit, which is where the case now rests. Should the appeals court also deny our standing, we will request review from the US Supreme Court.

In the midst of all this Pfizer changed the fellowship criteria, though everyone realizes that this was a way of evading the law while achieving the same desired result. The case is still active because of the disputed question of whether our anonymous member may serve as the lead plaintiff.

This is but one of several Do No Harm lawsuits in progress against governments, organizations, and programs that exclude people based on race. Other targets include the National Association of Emergency Medical Technicians, which offers a $1,250 "diversity scholarship" from which white students are barred from consideration—again, we are representing an anonymous student who is harmed by this racist provision—and the medical staffing agency Vituity, whose "Bridge to Brilliance" incentive program is offered solely to black physicians, who also receive a sign-up bonus of as much as $100,000.[166]

---

[166] "Do No Harm Sues National Association of Emergency Medical Technicians For Engaging In Racial Discrimination," Do No Harm, January 11, 2024; "Do No Harm Challenges Vituity's (CEP America LLC.) Racially Discriminatory Leadership Program," Do No Harm, December 11, 2023.

Sometimes companies and nonprofits scrap these unconstitutionally discriminatory programs in the blink of an eye. In June 2024, Do No Harm initiated a lawsuit against the American Association of University Women over a "Selected Professions Fellowship" that precluded white women from applying. A week later, the AAUW backed down, permitting white women to apply for the fellowship. (We shall see if any are chosen.)

The lesson to be drawn? As Dana Perino, former White House press secretary and current *Fox News* personality, says, "Watch out if Do No Harm shows up. They win their cases."

- - - - - -

Partnering with the Pacific Legal Foundation (PLF), Do No Harm has sued several states that discriminate on the basis of race in selecting members of various state medical boards.

These are flat-out violations of the Fourteenth Amendment to the US Constitution. Our cases are—or should be—slam dunks for justice.

For instance, a 2018 state law mandates that certain seats on the ten-member Louisiana State Board of Medical Examiners be reserved for racial minorities. Non-minority qualified potential board appointees may not even be considered for these seats. As I said at the time we filed the lawsuit, choosing candidates for a state medical board based on anything other than merit is corrosive to the mission and perception of the Louisiana State Board of Medical Examiners. Not only is this mandate grossly discriminatory, it also reflects the dangerous politicization of healthcare. Expertise and excellence are what matter, not skin color.

Montana, too, enshrouds its state Board of Medical Examiners in mandate madness, with the added twist of gender quotas. So the Big Sky State's unconstitutional law has also been targeted by Do No Harm and the Pacific Legal Foundation.

And we and our partners at PLF are trying to give the boot to a law in the Volunteer State that reserves at least one seat on the Tennessee

Board of Podiatric Medical Examiners for a racial minority. Qualified non-minority podiatrists are ineligible for this seat. The aforementioned cases are active and at various stages of court action.

These discriminatory laws are no fluky one-offs, nor are they exclusive to the medical field. A Pacific Legal Foundation Study, "Public Service Denied," found such unconstitutional race or sex-conscious mandates in twenty-five states, covering bodies ranging from the Arkansas Social Work Licensing Board to the Iowa State Judicial Nominating Commission. Do No Harm member Dr. Rodney Long Jr., the mental health therapist referenced earlier, has a private practice in Ohio and has been critical of the discriminatory requirement that the governor appoint to his state's Counselor, Social Worker, and Marriage and Family Therapist Board "at least one member...[who] shall be of African, Native American, Hispanic, or Asian descent."[167]

The problem isn't that African, Native American, Hispanic, or Asian therapists and social workers aren't deserving of membership on the board. Indeed, it would fine with Rodney (and Do No Harm) if racial minorities made up a majority or even the entirety of the board. All we ask is that health authorities focus solely on improving health outcomes, regardless of race, gender, or any other consideration. Fortunately, the Fourteenth Amendment agrees with us.

In this vein, I was questioned about our Louisiana lawsuit on an NPR program in New Orleans. I told the reporter that while we were suing because this was illegal discrimination, what bothered me most about the state's policy is that it was offensive to good minority physicians. Imagine, I said, if you were a black doctor who was appointed to the State Board of Medical Examiners because of your impressive achievements as one of the most respected members of a hospital staff or a community in the Pelican State. This ought to be a matter of justifiable

---

167 Laura D'Agostino and Angela C. Erickson, "Public Service Denied: How Discriminatory Mandates Prevent Qualified Individuals from Serving on Public Boards," Pacific Legal Foundation, October 2023.

pride. But instead, it causes embarrassment and frustration because deep down, you know that everyone thinks you have been chosen not for your considerable talents but merely on the basis of skin color.

This is terrible. Such laws undermine highly capable and respected physicians; they demean people who are worthy of admiration. But this is what you get when you racialize everything. Accomplished minority doctors are among the victims of DEI.

Oftentimes the mere filing of a lawsuit, or even the threat thereof, convinces the discriminating entity to rescind its policy. For instance, the Arkansas Minority Health Commission had offered a scholarship for students in the healthcare field that was only available to those of "African American, Hispanic, Native African/American Indian, Asian American or Marshallese" descent.

We filed suit against this outrageously illegal program in April 2023; by May, the Arkansas attorney general acknowledged its unconstitutionality, and the scholarship program was ended. The Arkansas pre-nursing student and Do No Harm member on whose behalf we filed the suit—"Member A," as her anonymous moniker had it—met all the scholarship's requirements...except she was the wrong color. Upon our victory she exulted, "Medical scholarships, like medicine itself, should be open to all. I am grateful that Arkansas ended its discrimination. Thank you to Do No Harm for helping me stand up for the Constitution and my rights."[168]

Working with the Pacific Legal Foundation, we have filed a lawsuit against the state of California for requiring physicians to take implicit bias training. This was the special project of a wonderful Do No Harm member, Dr. Marilyn Singleton: a black woman, an anesthesiologist, a third-generation physician, a tremendously impressive human being whose credo was, "I reject the unscientific accusation that people are defined by their race, not by their individual beliefs and choices."

---

[168] Do No Harm, "Arkansas Commission Ends Race Based Scholarship," press release, May 8, 2023.

Dr. Singleton was my colleague, my friend, my confidante, and a beacon in our fight for liberty and justice. She was such an inspiration. As a teenager, she protested California's Proposition 14, a 1964 ballot initiative that would have overturned a state fair housing act that banned sellers and landlords from discriminating when selling or renting accommodations. A passionate advocate of equal rights for African Americans, she boycotted Woolworth's segregated lunch counters. She was a fearless breaker of barriers, graduating from Stanford University and the University of California at San Francisco's medical school before beginning a storied career in medicine. While still practicing medicine, Marilyn attended UC Berkeley School of Law to gain a greater understanding of the intersection between public policy, law, and healthcare. She interned at the National Health Law Project and eventually practiced insurance and health law while maintaining her medical licenses and practice, all the time advocating tirelessly on behalf of her patients.

As DEI mandates began to sweep the nation, Dr. Singleton warned that a very ugly idea was experiencing a recrudescence: "DEI adherents are echoing the 1950s rhetoric of the opponents to integrated schools: people of different races learn better in separate environments where they can be their true selves. How is this diversity and inclusion?"[169]

Dr. Singleton adamantly refuted the false notion of implicit bias, calling it insulting and degrading to everyone involved in the practice and education of medicine. Never one to shy away from taking a public stand, she penned numerous op-eds, sat down for countless television interviews, hosted her own podcast, and cohosted our Do No Harm podcast.

In August 2023, Dr. Singleton and Do No Harm joined Dr. Azadeh Khatibi and the PLF in challenging a 2019 law that mandates implicit bias training as part of the required fifty hours of continuing medical education that all California physicians must log every two years as a condition of license renewal.

---

[169] Singleton, "Advocates for Equality Must Emerge from the Bunker and Speak Up."

Upon joining *Azadeh Khatibi, et al. v. Kristina Lawson, et. al,* Dr. Singleton declared, "The implicit bias requirement promotes the inaccurate belief that white individuals are naturally racist. This message can be detrimental to medical professionals and their patients as it creates an atmosphere of suspicion and animosity, which goes against the fundamental principle of doing no harm."[170]

The overkill in the California law exposed the nasty thought-control impulse at the heart of compulsory implicit bias courses. Attorney General Rob Bonta demanded to see a list of healthcare providers who had not yet taken implicit bias training—a clear intimidation tactic against independent thinkers.

Dr. Marilyn Singleton was one of the bravest and most independent thinkers I have ever known. Her death in June 2024 was occasion for mourning and it deepened our resolve to defend the principles she held so dearly.

Our energetic legal team is surely the most assiduous pen pal that the Office for Civil Rights in the US Department of Education has ever had.

As previously stated, you need standing—that is, the capacity to bring a lawsuit based on a plaintiff's connection to and harm from a challenged law—to sue Pfizer and other private, or ostensibly private, companies for discriminatory policies. By contrast, you don't need standing to sue public-university medical schools over race-based scholarships and the like. Typically, the policy in question is a fellowship targeting select racial minorities, and for which whites and perhaps Asians need not apply.

Medical schools and academic medical centers frequently offer visiting fellowships to bring in minority students in the hopes of recruiting

---

170   Do No Harm, "Do No Harm joins lawsuit to challenge California's mandatory implicit bias training in healthcare," press release, August 1, 2023.

them to their residency programs. The idea is that they will come in, see how nice it is to work there, and when it's time to graduate from medical school they will choose this as the place to do their training. There is one big problem, however: these fellowships often exclude those whose skin is the wrong hue.

You don't need standing to challenge these illegal programs. Anyone can do it, and the Office for Civil Rights will then launch an investigation. We are fortunate enough to work with Mark Perry, longtime professor of economics at the University of Michigan-Flint and a preternaturally diligent writer of letters to the DOE's OCR. (It's impossible to discuss these matters without lapsing into acronym-dropping.) Mark has issued well over two thousand such letters in his career. (I told you he was diligent!) Since Mark joined Do No Harm, he and our team have sent out upwards of 180 letters to the OCR, with many more to follow. As I write, fifty of these complaints have been opened for investigation, and a majority have been resolved in our favor.

Mark's philosophy is simple: "There is no 'good' form of discrimination, regardless of your intentions. It's all bad and illegal when you violate the law."

Ofttimes schools will immediately pull the fellowship upon receiving Do No Harm's complaint. For instance, when we brought one such to the attention of the University of Florida College of Medicine, its chief counsel told us that the med school had never consulted her. No one wants to deal with a federal agency investigation; UF dropped the discriminatory program.

On a parallel track with Do No Harm's legal challenges to DEI-distorted medicine, we are actively designing, publicizing, and lobbying for legislative solutions. In addition to the multiple state-level initiatives discussed in the previous chapter, Do No Harm is pursuing justice at the federal level as well.

Representative Greg Murphy (R-NC), a urologist who is the only practicing surgeon in Congress, has sponsored the EDUCATE Act, and we have been his partner every step of the way.

The bill, which at last count had more than sixty cosponsors, is predicated on the belief that DEI ideology is a danger to American medicine. So to restore medical education to its life-saving mission, Congressman Murphy's EDUCATE Act would eliminate *all* federal funding, including student loans, for medical schools that engage in the worst DEI practices. Schools would have to agree to the following:

— *No racist teaching*. Medical schools teach about "intersectionality," "colonization," and "white supremacy" while promoting the idea that people are either "oppressors" or "oppressed." These concepts push medical students to treat patients differently based on race, sex or "gender identity"—as the head of Brigham and Women's Hospital in Boston did by proposing preferential treatment for "Black and Latinx heart failure patients."

— *No racial discrimination*. Medical schools increasingly offer scholarships, classes, and programming designed for—and sometimes available only to—students of specific races. This includes "affinity groups" students can join voluntarily, as well as classes that segregate students for the sake of learning.

— *No loyalty oaths*. Medical schools routinely require applicants and faculty to write DEI statements as a condition of acceptance or employment. Such requirements violate freedom of speech and eviscerate merit. Schools reject candidates for not mouthing progressive platitudes while choosing others for their devotion to DEI.

— *No DEI offices*. Most medical schools have a department, team, or office dedicated to DEI. These bureaucracies exist to spread a divisive ideology across campus, from the curriculum to extracurricular activities.

In addition to denying federal money to schools that engage in these practices, the EDUCATE Act would prevent accrediting organizations, such as the Liaison Committee on Medical Education and the Association of American Medical Colleges, from requiring DEI education at medical schools.[171]

Federal and state monies are the lifeblood of the DEI regime in medical schools and organizations. It's time to stanch the flow.

- - - - - -

The original Hippocratic Oath spoke of treating all patients, no matter what their social station, equally and with the utmost skill of the physician. We need to rededicate ourselves to this high standard and to guarantee that we will not propagandize to our patients or attempt to indoctrinate them but will only see them as God's children who turn to us for comfort and, we hope, cure. We must also guarantee to the American people that we will dedicate ourselves to training the most meritorious individuals as the physicians who will have the privilege of caring for these patients. Anything less will tarnish the respect and trust that our profession has earned over the centuries and must continue to enjoy in the future.

The best way to do no harm is to do good medicine.

Yet medical people are afraid. They fear retribution for expressing their honest (and entirely defensible) opinions. This is a sad reality in what we call, before every sporting event, the "land of the free and the home of the brave," but there you are.

Things have gotten somewhat better, or less Stalinist, over the last three years. The Red Guards–level hateful rage against dissenters has calmed, to an extent. The gestalt of that academic world in roughly the years 2016–2022 was truly frightening.

---

[171] Greg Murphy and Stanley Goldfarb, "Ban DEI Quackery in Medical Schools," *Wall Street Journal*, March 18, 2024; US Congressman Gregory F. Murphy, MD, "Murphy Introduces Bill to Ban DEI in Medicine," press release, March 19, 2024.

Now and then a fellow member of, say, my dinner club for senior medical people will whisper a word of agreement or encouragement to me, but this is *sotto voce*. I guess an open endorsement of my opinions is too professionally and personally risky.

But I won't be silenced. Nor will Do No Harm.

As the provocative social critic Andrew Sullivan concluded in December 2023:

> End DEI in its entirety. Fire all the administrators whose only job is to enforce its toxic orthodoxy. Admit students on academic merit alone. Save standardized testing—which in fact helps minorities, and it's "the best way to distinguish smart poor kids from stupid rich kids," as Steven Pinker said this week. Restore grading so that it actually means something again. Expel students who shut or shout down speech or deplatform speakers. Pay no attention to the race or sex or orientation or gender identity of your students, and see them as free human beings with open minds. Treat them equally as individuals seeking to learn, if you can remember such a concept.[172]

Is diversity the most important factor in recruitment and hiring for pilots? What about neurosurgeons? There are certain societal roles where merit and only merit should be the basis for entry.

Physician is at the top of that list. Let's keep it that way.

172   Andrew Sullivan, "The Day the Empress' Clothes Fell Off," *The Weekly Dish*, December 8, 2023, https://andrewsullivan.substack.com/p/the-day-the-empress-clothes-fell-ffa.

CHAPTER SIX

ALL ABOARD THE TRANS TRAIN?

How did Do No Harm, which began by taking on DEI and identity politics in medicine, transition—if you will forgive the verb—into the childhood gender treatment field as well?

It started when we spoke to early donors who felt strongly that this was a particularly egregious—and dangerous—form of identity politics. Some of them had children or loved ones who had traveled partway or even all the way down this path, and that was a real motivating factor.

The issue wasn't on my radar, though I was aware of the health concerns of transgender adults. When I was at Penn a gay student asked if we could have a day devoted to gay and transgender medicine. I thought it was a good idea. So we had faculty involved in the field give talks about the special challenges of caring for gay and transgender patients. No big deal.

But childhood gender transition is a whole other matter. A deep dive into the issue radicalized me. This is a terrible development that will ruin the lives of tens, even hundreds of thousands of our fellow

Americans who are making life-defining decisions before they are capable of informed consent.

The two issues—DEI and childhood gender transition—are connected in that both are manifestations of identity politics. Confused kids are told by counselors or doctors at gender clinics that they are trans, and all of a sudden they belong to an oppressed category. They are victims. Their individuality is erased; they must all be treated the same.

Nowhere is the Hippocratic injunction to do no harm more important than in the care of our children and teenagers, which is why the organization that takes its name from this sacred motto is fighting to curtail the unscientific and individually harmful practice of so-called "gender-affirming care."

(Before we go further, a note on terminology. I never write "gender-affirming care" without either prefacing it with "so-called" or placing it within doubt-indicating quotation marks. People practicing such "care" are not affirming the child's gender but rather subverting it.)

"Gender-affirming care" is based on the dangerous premise that *any child* experiencing distress that he or she thinks is related to his or her sex should automatically be placed on the conveyor belt of gender transition. This begins with social transitioning to the sexual identity of their choice, is followed by puberty blockers, then cross-sex hormones, and finally, in some cases, radical surgery to remove healthy body parts. The middle two steps are almost seamless: multiple studies show that virtually all (98 percent in one widely cited survey) children who start on puberty blockers "graduate" to cross-sex hormones.[173]

A vastly disproportionate number of gender-confused minors are anxious, depressed, autistic, or suffering from eating or personality disorders, but underlying emotional or mental health problems are seldom

---

[173] See, for instance, Polly Carmichael et al., "Short-term outcomes of pubertal suppression in a selected cohort of 12 to 15 year old young people with persistent gender dysphoria in the UK," *PLOS ONE*, February 2, 2021.

addressed by the typical gender clinic.[174] Even self-harming behavior and suicidal ideation do not stand in the way of children receiving permanent disfiguring and sterilizing treatments. Dr. Diana Tordoff, often cited in her support of giving cross-sex hormones to teenagers, has admitted that patients at Seattle Children's Hospital's gender clinic who have "depression, anxiety, or suicidal thoughts" are "not precluded access" to treatments.[175]

There are clinics that put kids on puberty blockers and hormone treatments without any psychiatric referrals as long as the parents consent. There's not even the pretense of an evaluation to determine if the child is depressed, autistic, has been abused, or has any of the usual markers.

The refusal to approach each child on an individual basis is reason enough to oppose the movement toward "gender-affirming care."

Yet there's another reason it deserves criticism: the impossibility of informed consent by the minors who are subjected to this treatment. Young children and adolescents are inappropriately being allowed to make potentially irreversible life-altering decisions, in many cases without parental consent or engagement.

These procedures can lead to impairment in bone strength and brain maturation, loss of fertility and the ability to engage in sexual relations, and adherence to a lifelong pharmaceutical regimen. Yet puberty blockers have been prescribed in the United States to minor patients as young as eight!

It is dangerous, destructive, and grossly irresponsible to let children, whose minds are still developing, make such life-altering decisions at such young ages—especially since 90 percent of children who believe they are a different sex no longer hold that view as adults if they are left to develop on their own, without medical interventions.

---

[174]   The best numbers we have on this phenomenon suggest that about 30 percent of the young people in gender clinics are autistic.

[175]   Stanley Goldfarb and Dr. Miriam Grossman, "Even progressive Europe won't go as far as America in child transgender treatments," *New York Post*, January 30, 2023.

Moreover, as we shall see, "gender-affirming care" balances precariously on an ultra-thin evidentiary foundation. A glaring lack of scientific research undergirds it.

Activists make up for the absence of solid evidence by squelching debate, spreading misinformation, bullying those who express doubts, and seeking to discredit actual scientific evidence detailing the risks of childhood gender transition.

From a medical standpoint, the misuse of the literature on this subject is deeply disturbing. No one has documented any real benefit from childhood transition. Of course, in any study there are outliers at each end of the distribution: a few are better off, a few meet with total disaster. But you can't assist in these transitions without knowing which kids will benefit and which will suffer. To do so is profoundly irresponsible. We have no clear understanding of the criteria by which to judge if a transitioned child will grow into a fulfilled and competent adult or a complete mess. Yet the medical and gender establishment in the US is exposing them to drugs and even performing radical surgeries upon these children at a time when they really can't make informed decisions!

I restrict this criticism to the United States because in recent years, as trustworthy physicians have scrutinized the literature and evidence, many European nations have come to the conclusion that childhood gender transition should either be severely restricted or altogether banned.

"Gender affirmation," the current American approach to transgender medical treatment for children, insists that questioning a minor's gender self-definition is harmful and unethical. The American Academy of Pediatrics has embraced an affirm-only/affirm-early policy since 2018, despite withering medical and scientific criticism.[176] "Gender-affirming care," with no or minimal questions asked of gender dysphoric minors before beginning treatment, remains the standard across most of the United States.

---

[176] Jason Rafferty et al., "Ensuring Comprehensive Care and Support for Transgender and Gender-Diverse Children and Adolescents," *Pediatrics* 142, no. 4 (2018).

Do No Harm is committed to ensuring that children who believe they have gender identity disorder are treated with the utmost care, caution, and concern. We fight to protect children, assert truth, and defend science.

- - - - - -

I will say at the outset that it's possible that there are children who will benefit from transitioning. The problem is that we do not know and currently have no way of knowing who they are.

Gender dysphoria is real but rare. The classic cases are those children who feel from a very young age that they are the "wrong" sex. They cross-dress or desire to do so from the start. The boys want to wear dresses, and the girls can't stand long hair.

We do not know if this is a condition of the body or the mind. Biology is very complicated, and some genetic traits do govern behavior. There is no question that there are transgender adults who are better off for having undergone transitioning. But we really have no idea how to determine who will profit and who will suffer from transitioning, and minors are simply too young to make so momentous a decision on the spur of the moment.

Today, the number of diagnosed or asserted cases of gender dysphoria dwarfs those of the past. Almost all these new cases differ radically from the classic cases. They exhibited no signs of gender dysphoria as young children; rather, these feelings swept over them at the age of twelve or thirteen or fourteen. They discovered their alleged dysphoria around the time of puberty. They are, in the main, adolescent girls with a variety of psychological comorbidities.

These children may meet some resistance when first informing their parents of this epiphany, but eventually their parents take them to a pediatrician, who sends them to a gender clinic, where advocates of "gender-affirming care" tell the children that yes, they were born the wrong gender, and tell the parents that if they do not offer their offspring whole-heartedly uncritical support the kids might well commit suicide. A child taking his or her own life is a parent's worst nightmare, so the parent ceases resistance and goes all-in on the transition. Meanwhile, the kids, riding the fad, get to act out in the dual role of victims and heroes.

What these children need more than anything is a good psychiatric examination. Yet incredibly, no one ever gives most of these children an in-depth psychiatric evaluation, which was once *de rigueur* for patients professing gender dysphoria.

Dr. Jason Rafferty, lead author of "Ensuring Comprehensive Care and Support for Transgender and Gender-Diverse Children and Adolescents," the American Academy of Pediatrics' policy statement on gender care for minors, has said that "the child's sense of reality and feeling of who they are is the navigational beacon to sort of orient treatment around."[177] This is preposterous. If a patient comes into a physician's office and informs the doctor that he feels as though he has a broken wrist or lung cancer or eczema or any of a thousand diseases or disorders, the doctor will listen respectfully and then apply his or her training and expertise, combined with the latest medical technology, to make a professional diagnosis that may or may not confirm the patient's suspicion. But this is so yesteryear, a relic of the benighted Stone Age, when it comes to gender dysphoria among minors, at least in Dr. Rafferty's astonishingly unscientific formulation. The child knows best, and the job of the physician or therapist is to shape the treatment around "the child's sense of reality and feeling of who they are."

Detransitioner Hacsi Horvath, an epidemiologist who lectures in the Department of Epidemiology and Biostatistics at the University of California, San Francisco, has written that young people who believe they suffer from gender dysphoria "typically only visit doctors and psychotherapists who are willing (or even eager) to 'affirm' their opinion

---

[177] Leor Sapir, "The reckoning over puberty blockers has arrived," *The Hill*, April 4, 2024; Rafferty et al., "Ensuring Comprehensive Care and Support for Transgender and Gender-Diverse Children and Adolescents."

that they are somehow inhabiting the wrong body." They come for a rubber stamp and that's what they get. It's as if a child comes into a physician's office, announces that he has diabetes, and is given insulin—without ever doing a lab test!

Horvath adds that "persons in the driven, obsessed stages of gender dysphoria can seemingly think of nothing except transition. No-one dreams of asking them to slow down, to seek psychotherapy, perhaps even find a way through this work to prevent transition, which can be costly on so many levels." Young people get green lights all the way, only to find at the end of the journey that there is no road back.[178] (Per Mr. Horvath, a "detransitioner" is one who ceases or even seeks to reverse the effects of transgender treatments. More on them anon.)

Forty or fifty years ago, pre-internet, a child confused about his or her gender would go to a parent, a counselor, or a doctor, and—one hopes—find a sympathetic ear but also a voice advising to proceed with caution, to work through this. Psychiatrists practiced what they called "watchful waiting," in which psychiatric therapy and time, the great healer, would usually relieve the patient of the desire to change his or her sex.

Today, the child goes online immediately to one-sided websites that shill for transition, presenting it as the solution to every problem. Caution is for old fogeys; the old practice of "wait and watch" is derided as kinder, gentler transphobia. It's all systems go and damn the torpedoes. Advocates—most of whom are sincere, I believe, although captive of an ideology—affirm, affirm, and affirm, creating an echo chamber of unstinting and unquestioning support for each stage of a child's transformation from boy into pretend girl and vice versa.

The transsexual-industrial complex, by contrast, is sincere only in the sense that it sincerely wishes to maximize profits. The number of

---

[178] Hacsi Horvath, "The Theatre of the Body: A detransitioned epidemiologist examines suicidality, affirmation, and transgender identity," 4thWaveNow, December 19, 2018.

177

pediatric gender clinics in the United States has exploded from zero in 2007 to over one hundred today.[179]

The amount spent on transitioning minors is enormous. The transgender journey is expensive; in current dollars, it's a lifetime commitment of half a million dollars or more. In 2015, researchers at the Johns Hopkins Bloomberg School of Public Health found that for those choosing surgery, healthcare costs were between $34,000 and $43,000 over the first five years, gradually falling to $7,000–$10,000 per year after ten years. Thus, a teen who transitions and lives his or her appointed three score and ten years will incur perhaps $750,000 in trans-related medical expenses.[180]

Among Do No Harm's signature features is our Stop the Harm database, which measures the cost and extent of the sex-change industry and the financial windfall it provides to its promoters.

Do No Harm looked at the transgender medical interventions (puberty blockers, cross-sex hormones, and surgeries) performed on minors at children's hospitals and affiliated health systems between 2019 and 2023. The facilities for which there are publicly available data provided nearly fourteen thousand treatments (including 5,700 surgeries) at a total cost to insurance companies and taxpayers of nearly $120 million. The real numbers are almost certainly much higher, since major health systems such as Kaiser Permanente don't disclose data, nor do patients who pay out of pocket.[181]

These numbers barely hint at the bonanza this industry is in for if we don't put an end to the exploitation of these children. They merely suggest the immensity of this business opportunity, for each child ensnared in this web will be a customer for life. Despite barely existing before

[179] Chad Terhune, Robin Respaut, and Michelle Conlin, "As more transgender children seek medical care, families confront many unknowns," Reuters, October 6, 2022.

[180] "Study: Paying for Transgender Health Care Cost-Effective," Johns Hopkins Bloomberg School of Public Health, December 1, 2015, https://publichealth.jhu.edu/2015/study-paying-for-transgender-health-care-cost-effective.

[181] Stanley Goldfarb and Roy Eappen, "Money Is Driving Medicine's Embrace of Child Transgenderism," *National Review*, October 14, 2024.

2018, gender transitions for children will likely soon be a billion-dollar industry, if they aren't already. It has been estimated that transgender surgeries alone, across all age groups, will generate $5 billion by 2030.[182]

Do No Harm's analysis reveals that the average intervention makes more than $8,500 for medical providers. That's significantly more than the cost of the typical hospital stay, which, according to provider MDC Healthcare, averages $2,600 per day in the US.[183] All told, the cost of the average transgender treatment for a child is equivalent to 62 percent of annual healthcare spending per person, based on federal data.[184] In other words, hospitals and health systems can bill most of a patient's annual medical expenses in a single day.

Transgender medicine for children is potentially a jackpot—if a deeply corrupted one. The Children's Hospital of Los Angeles opened its transgender center in 2015 and billed $1.5 million in surgeries alone between 2019 and 2023.

Incredibly, Children's Hospital of Los Angeles is not even among the top ten billing institutions for sex-change treatments for minors. This Wall of Shame reads:

1—Mount Sinai Medical Center (New York City)

2—Boston Children's Hospital (Boston, MA)

3—Surgery Center of Texas, LP (Plano, TX)

4—Lucile Packard Children's Hospital Stanford (Palo Alto, CA)

5—Legacy Good Samaritan Medical Center (Portland, OR)

6—New York University (New York City)

7—Center for Advanced Plastic Surgery, Inc. (Thousand Oaks, CA)

8—Hospital of the University of Pennsylvania (Philadelphia, PA)

---

[182]   Ben Zeisloft, "Transgender Surgery Poised To Become A $5 Billion Industry," *The Daily Wire*, October 4, 2022.

[183]   "Understanding the Cost of In-Home Care and the Cost of a Hospital Stay," MDC Healthcare, https://www.mdchealthcare.org/, accessed October 28, 2024.

[184]   "National health expenditure data," Centers for Medicare & Medicaid Services, https://www.cms.gov/data-research/statistics-trends-and-reports/national-health-expenditure-data/historical, accessed October 28, 2024.

9—University Hospital (Ann Arbor, MI)

10—Alderwood Surgery Center, LLC (Lynnwood, WA)

For the most in-depth look at who is making a fortune off trans treatments for children, please visit Do No Harm's "Stop the Harm" website at https://stoptheharmdatabase.com.

- - - - - -

The belief that biological sex and gender are socially constructed has made its way into American classrooms, courtrooms, bathrooms, and boardrooms. The mainstreaming of this belief system has coincided with a substantial increase in the under-eighteen population receiving transgender medical care. Between 2017 and 2021, the number of children known to be on puberty blockers or cross-sex hormones more than doubled.[185] Over that same period, the number of youths age seventeen and under diagnosed with gender dysphoria almost tripled, from 15,172 to 42,167.[186]

Skeptics have pointed out that the surge in gender interventions (i.e., social transformation, puberty blockers, cross-sex hormones, and sex reassignment surgeries) might be explained, at least in part, by social contagion. According to this argument, the increase in interventions for adolescents is caused not by an authentic increase in the incidence of gender incongruence but by the spread of gender ideology across all facets of American life. This concern is exacerbated by the degree to which the medical establishment allows such ideology to compete with or even usurp the scientific method as a guide to research and medical practice.

Is the explosion of gender dysphoria a social contagion, a la the Salem Witch Trials, or is it just that young people are only now realizing that changing one's secondary sex characteristics is an option? I do not say

---

[185] Chad Terhune, Robin Respaut, and Michelle Conlin, "As more transgender children seek medical care, families confront many unknowns."

[186] Robin Respaut and Chad Terhune, "Putting numbers on the rise in children seeking gender care," Reuters, October 6, 2022.

"changing one's sex" because that is impossible. A man who takes estrogen, grows breasts, has his sex organs removed, and even receives a fake vagina is still a man—even if the Columbia University Vagelos College of Physicians & Surgeons instructs med students to say "people with uteruses" instead of "women" with reference to that female organ.[187]

The gender dysphorics today are lopsidedly female, and, as mentioned, frequently they are beset by anxiety, depression, and various personality disorders. They are, quite possibly, part of a social contagion. Treading carefully in the pages of *Psychology Today*, Dr. Robert Bartholomew writes:

> It sounds sexist, and it's sure to raise the ire of some feminists, but the literature does not lie. Throughout history, groups of people in cohesive social units have suddenly fallen ill or exhibited strange behaviors, from headaches and fainting spells to twitching, shaking, and trance states. But whether it's an outbreak of spirit possession at a shoe factory in Malaysia, a collapsing marching band at a school gala in England, or a twitching epidemic in a Louisiana high school, the pattern is invariably the same. Most, and often all of those affected, are females. In fact, of the 2,000+ cases in my files that date back to 1566, this pattern holds true over 99 percent of the time.[188]

(Do No Harm takes no position on the etiology of the current gender dysphoria explosion. But Dr. Bartholomew's is an interesting point.)

---

[187] "Guidelines for Promoting an Anti-Bias and Inclusive Curriculum," Columbia University Vagelos College of Physicians & Surgeons, https://www.vagelos.columbia. edu/education/academic-programs/md-program/curriculum/guidelines-promoting-anti-bias-and-inclusive-curriculum.

[188] Robert Bartholomew, "Why Are Females Prone to Mass Hysteria?" *Psychology Today*, March 31, 2017.

Physician-researcher Dr. Lisa Littman, formerly of the Brown University School of Public Health and now Director of the Institute for Comprehensive Gender Dysphoria Research, coined the term "rapid-onset gender dysphoria" (ROGD) to describe the "phenomenon whereby teens and young adults who did not exhibit childhood signs of gender issues appeared to suddenly identify as transgender."

She explained to Jonathan Kay of *Quillette* that she "became interested in studying gender dysphoria when I observed, in my own community, an unusual pattern whereby teens from the same friend group began announcing transgender identities on social media, one after the other, on a scale that greatly exceeded expected numbers. I searched online and found several narratives of parents describing this type of pattern happening with their teen and young adult kids who had no history of gender dysphoria during their childhoods.... Then, I spoke with a clinician who was hearing her clients describe this phenomenon as something happening in their families. The descriptions of multiple friends from the same pre-existing group becoming transgender-identified at the same time were very surprising. Parents reported that, after announcing a transgender identity, the kids became increasingly sullen, withdrawn and hostile toward their families. They also said that the clinicians they saw were only interested in fast-tracking gender-affirmation and transition and were resistant to even evaluating the child's pre-existing and current mental health issues."[189]

In 2018, Dr. Littman published what became an explosive study of ROGD in the journal *PLOS ONE*. She posted a ninety-question survey to websites on which parents had reported that their child had experienced a rapid onset of gender dysphoria during or after puberty.

Parents completed 256 surveys. The vast majority of their gender dysphoric children (82.8 percent) were female, and the mean age for all children at the time of their transgender identification was 15.2

---

[189] Jonathan Kay, "An Interview With Lisa Littman, Who Coined the Term 'Rapid Onset Gender Dysphoria,'" *Quillette*, March 19, 2019.

years. More than two in five (41 percent) of the children had a non-heterosexual orientation before identifying as transgender. More than three in five (62.5 percent) had been diagnosed with "at least one mental health disorder or neurodevelopmental disability prior to the onset of their gender dysphoria," and 69.4 percent of respondents said that their adolescent had social anxiety. Nearly half had been harming themselves through cutting or other non-suicidal self-injury. None of the minors in the study "would have met diagnostic criteria for gender dysphoria in childhood."

Parents had noted significant changes in their children's behavior since the transgender identification. They reported declines in their children's mental health (47.2 percent of survey respondents), worsening of parent-child relationships (57.3 percent), the child isolating himself or herself from the family (46.6 percent), expressing distrust of non-transgender people (22.7 percent), and no longer spending time with non-transgender friends (25 percent). In about two-thirds of cases (63.8 percent), the child had called a parent a transphobe or bigot.[190]

In 86.7 percent of cases, explained Dr. Littman in an interview, "This new identification seemed to occur in the context of either belonging to a group of friends [in which] multiple—or even all—members became transgender-identified around the same time, or through immersion in social media, or both."[191] The social media sites most often cited by parents as being influential in their child's perceived metamorphosis were YouTube (63.6 percent) and Tumblr (61.7 percent).

In one striking case, four young teenaged girls who were taking lessons from a popular coach announced that they were transgender after the coach came out as transgender.

---

[190] Lisa Littman, "Parent reports of adolescents and young adults perceived to show signs of a rapid onset of gender dysphoria," *PLOS ONE* 14, no. 3 (August 16, 2018; correction March 19, 2019).

[191] Kay, "An Interview With Lisa Littman, Who Coined the Term 'Rapid Onset Gender Dysphoria.'"

The parental respondents were hardly the foaming transphobes who haunt activists' imaginations. Though concerned about their children's sudden transgender identity, they were overwhelmingly in favor of gay marriage (85.9 percent approval), for instance. But over three-quarters (76.5 percent) believed their child was incorrectly identifying as transgender.

Dr. Littman raised the possibility that the rapid-onset phenomenon could be the result of peer or social contagion. She noted that "social contagion is the spread of affect or behaviors through a population. Peer contagion, in particular, is the process where an individual and peer mutually influence each other in a way that promotes emotions and behaviors that can potentially have negative effects on their development." She added that peer contagion "has been associated with depressive symptoms, disordered eating, aggression, bullying, and drug use."[192]

Adding weight to the social contagion explanation is that in the past, gender dysphoria developed in isolation rather than as part of a group phenomenon. It wasn't contagious; its development in one person had no connection to the experience of others.[193]

With respect to eating disorders, Dr. Littman explained that in treatment settings for those suffering anorexia nervosa, "there is a group dynamic where the 'best' anorexics (those who are thinnest, most resistant to gaining weight, and who have experienced the most medical complications from their disease) are admired, validated, and seen as authentic while the patients who want to recover from anorexia and cooperate with medical treatment are maligned, ridiculed, and marginalized.... If similar mechanisms are at work in the context of gender dysphoria, this greatly complicates" evaluation and treatment.

---

[192] Littman, "Parent reports of adolescents and young adults perceived to show signs of a rapid onset of gender dysphoria."
[193] Shrier, *Irreversible Damage: The Transgender Craze Seducing Our Daughters*, 133.

Eighteen is not a magic number but that's what society seems to have agreed is the age of maturity. Raheem Williams, a senior fellow at Do No Harm, says: "It's a fundamental question: What exactly is a minor? Why do we have legal protections for minors? That's what we need to think about right now. I live in a country where you must be 21 to buy cigarettes but I'm being told that even a 12-year-old can understand the ramifications of a sex change."

I am a strong First Amendment person. I would not censor the websites that push trans on young people nor would I punish those who publish on them. Alas, many on the other side would censor us without a moment's thought. Too many woke activists are "free speech for me but not for thee" hypocrites.

However, regulating the activities of children is a legitimate governmental function. Drinking, smoking, viewing pornography, drug-taking: these are within the purview of the law, and their effects—unlike gender transition—are not (typically) irreversible.

Look: I don't give a damn if an adult wishes to take hormones or have his or her body radically altered—mutilated, perhaps—to fulfill his desire to "be" the other sex. But do not start confused children down this road. Within five years of social transitioning, perhaps 60 percent of children will be on puberty blockers and/or cross-sex hormones.[194] In almost all cases, puberty blockers lead to cross-sex hormones, and about one in three transgender-identifying persons will eventually chose surgery, which may include having their breasts removed or penises inverted into fake vaginas.[195] (Radical bottom surgery is a bridge too far for many of the women who seek to transition. While 61 percent

---

[194]   Kristina R. Olson et al., "Gender Identity 5 Years After Social Transition," *Pediatrics* 150, no. 2 (2022).

[195]   Ian T. Nolan et al., "Demographic and temporal trends in transgender identities and gender confirming surgery," *Translational Andrology and Urology* 8, no. 3 (June 2019): 184–190.

of women who identify as trans men desire top surgery, and 36 percent have had it, just 13 percent desire phalloplasty, and only 3 percent have gone through with it.[196])

Transitioning is a train from which, once you reach a certain point, you are not allowed to disembark.

That is why Do No Harm opposes "social transitioning" for minors. One particular harm of social transitioning is that it is not infrequently done behind parental backs. School counselors, nurses, and gender activists collude with the child by giving him or her a chest binder, a tuck-friendly swimsuit to conceal male genitals, or even a new name that is used in school but without the knowledge of mom or dad.

The Massachusetts Department of Elementary and Secondary Education has actually established a policy of enforced parental ignorance. It states:

> Some transgender and gender nonconforming students are not openly so at home for reasons such as safety concerns or lack of acceptance. School personnel should speak with the student first before discussing a student's gender nonconformity or transgender status with the student's parent or guardian. For the same reasons, school personnel should discuss with the student how the school should refer to the student, e.g., appropriate pronoun use, in written communication to the student's parent or guardian.[197]

Apparently bureaucrats know better than mom and dad what is best for a child.

California has a law that "protects" children claiming gender dysphoria from parents who may not be gung-ho for name changes, absurd

---

[196] Shrier, *Irreversible Damage: The Transgender Craze Seducing Our Daughters*, 177.
[197] "Guidance for Massachusetts Public Schools Creating a Safe and Supportive School Environment," Massachusetts Department of Elementary and Secondary Education, https://www.doe.mass.edu/sfs/lgbtq/genderidentity.html, accessed September 20, 2024.

pronouns, chest binding, penis tucking, and the rest of the routine. Signed into law by Governor Gavin Newsom in July 2024, the Orwellian-named SAFETY (Support Academic Futures and Educators for Today's Youth) Act outlaws "parental notification policies that require teachers to inform parents if their child asks to use a name or pronoun different than what was assigned at birth, or if they engage in activities and use spaces designed for the opposite sex." The law was a heavy-handed response to seven California school districts that had put such parental notification policies in place.[198]

These children need to be seen by a psychiatrist, who can discover what conflicts or traumas have led to this moment. Do not bind a twelve-year-old's breasts! Detransitioners often speak of the pain caused by breast binding. As Abigail Shrier says, "It turns out that breasts—glandular tissue, fatty tissue, blood vessels, lymph vessels and lymph nodes, lobes, ducts, connective tissue, and ligaments—are not really meant to be squashed flat all day long."[199] Not only does abetting the delusion that one has been born the wrong sex do a monumental disservice to the great majority of these kids, who will eventually accept their birth sex, but it also hurts like hell.

Once ensconced in the cocoon of gender affirmation, the child will be started on drugs. These make him or her feel better—it is what she wants, after all—and the parents feel better, too, because their son or daughter does not hate them anymore. In the near term, many of these children will say they are happy. The real question, though, is what happens five or ten years down the line, when the irreversible effects of what has been done sink in, fully and finally?

---

[198] Diana Lambert, "California law prohibits schools from requiring staff to reveal students' gender identity," EdSource, July 16, 2024. California has also been a "leader," if that is not abusing that noun, in the mandatory pronoun movement. In 2017, Governor Jerry Brown signed into law a measure authorizing punishment—up to and including jail time—for healthcare workers in hospitals, nursing homes, and assisted living facilities who "willfully and repeatedly" refuse to use a transgender person's "preferred name or pronouns." Brooke Singman, "New California law allows jail time for using wrong gender pronoun, sponsor denies that would happen," Fox News, October 9, 2017.

[199] Shrier, *Irreversible Damage: The Transgender Craze Seducing Our Daughters*, 47.

Going through puberty is healthy; delaying or denying it has serious physical, mental, and emotional consequences. To quote the American College of Pediatricians, "Puberty is not a disease. It is a critical window of normal development that is radically disrupted by puberty blockers like Lupron. When normal puberty is arrested, valuable time is forever stolen from these children, time during which significant advances in bone, brain, sexual and psycho-social development occur; time that can never be given back."[200]

Puberty blockers are drugs that bind to the pituitary gland. They mimic the normal hormones that the pituitary gland would put out to signal sex organs such as the ovaries and testicles to make the hormones that convey the secondary sex characteristics. These blockers bind to the same receptor but tell the pituitary that it has already made enough of these hormones. The gland stops pumping them out and thereby blocks the surge of the hormones that enable pubertal development.

These may sound like Dr. Frankenstein potions but they have a respectable provenance. In rare cases children begin puberty prematurely, and these drugs delay the onset to a more appropriate time in the child's young life.

Puberty blockers are typically taken for three or four years: the length of puberty. These are often administered in the form of a drug called LUPRON DEPOT-PED, which is injected in the child's arm or under the skin and released slowly.

LUPRON, which before the recent avalanche of gender dysphoria cases had typically been prescribed for the small number of young patients with precocious puberty, has some nasty physical and psychiatric effects. According to the drug's manufacturer, these include vaginal

200   "Deconstructing Transgender Pediatrics," American College of Pediatricians, https://acpeds.org/topics/sexuality-issues-of-youth/gender-confusion-and-transgender-identity/deconstructing-transgender-pediatrics, accessed September 15, 2024.

bleeding and "symptoms of emotional liability, such as crying, irritability, impatience, anger, and aggression."[201]

In addition to mood disorders, the use of LUPRON, even temporarily, has been associated with cognitive impairment, osteoporosis, and seizures.[202] As a side note, the drug is also used to treat prostate cancer and breast cancer—and as a means of chemically castrating sex offenders.

Bicalutamide, which treats prostate cancer by blocking the effect of the male hormone androgen, is also prescribed as a puberty blocker. It feminizes boys, assisting in the growth of breasts. Its unpleasant side effects, which are almost too long to list, include, most portentously, liver toxicity.[203]

The problem with blocking puberty is that puberty is essential to normal maturation of a human being. As the American College of Pediatricians says, it is necessary to brain and bone development. Although there is no conclusive evidence either way, it seems that bypassing puberty may have negative effects on cognitive and psychological development. It also appears related to abnormal bone function, which leads to increased incidence of bone fractures and osteoporosis later in life.[204]

Dr. Sally Baxendale, professor of clinical neuropsychology at the University College of London, says that "blocking puberty prevents the critical rewiring in the brain that underpins the ability make complex decisions. Puberty blockers may give children time to think but they simultaneously rob them of their developing capacity to do so."[205]

A recent Mayo Clinic study suggested that puberty blockers may have irreversible effects on fertility. Atrophied testicles and stunted sperm production cells were found in a sample of ten-to-sixteen-year-old boys—nine of whom were on puberty blockers—who claimed a trans

---

[201] "LUPRON DEPOT-PED," lupronped.com.

[202] "Deconstructing Transgender Pediatrics," American College of Pediatricians.

[203] "Bicalutamide," NIH National Library of Medicine, https://medlineplus.gov/druginfo/meds/a697047.html.

[204] "The Effect of Puberty Blockers on the Accrual of Bone Mass," Society for Evidence Based Gender Medicine, May 1, 2021, https://segm.org/.

[205] Sapir, "The reckoning over puberty blockers has arrived."

identity. The researchers raised the possibility that the harm to testicular development may be permanent.[206] Although puberty blockers are sold as a "pause" in development, it may not be possible to pick up, developmentally, where one left off.

(Incidentally, women who transition as adults find that undergoing normal puberty is no bar to appearing masculine. Post-pubertal women who take high doses of testosterone become very masculinized; they grow facial hair and take on a male appearance. However, it's harder for men. If they do not take female sex hormones during puberty they will not look terribly feminine as adults. Waiting until eighteen is fine for girls but, to be honest, not for boys. But we do know that the vast majority of these boys will shed their gender dysphoria as adults and live as men—often gay men.)

Puberty having been blocked, the next step is to administer the hormones associated with the opposite sex. (That phrase—*opposite sex*—is enough to get the unwary canceled in most American medical schools.) Virtually every young person who goes on puberty blockers graduates into sex hormone therapy.

In hormone treatment, the child patient is given large doses of estrogen if male and testosterone if female. These produce secondary sex characteristics: the men will grow large breasts, which can be augmented by surgery, and the women will grow facial hair and a masculine musculature. Their voices will also change.

The impact on the secondary sex characteristics is deleterious. If women are exposed to high doses of testosterone their epithelium will develop abnormally, leading to urinary problems and chronic pain. A study in the *International Urogynecology Journal* found that 94 percent of a sample of sixty-eight trans-identified female patients—what the authors refer to as "transgender men"—on hormone therapy had pelvic

---

[206] James Reinl, "Puberty blockers may NOT be reversible and could raise children's risk of fertility problems and even cancer, Mayo Clinic study suggests," *Daily Mail*, April 5, 2024.

floor dysfunction and 87 percent exhibited urinary incontinence or other urinary symptoms. As if that weren't enough, 53 percent suffered from sexual dysfunction and 45 percent had anorectal symptoms.[207]

The young girls chatting blithely on trans-friendly websites about "T" (testosterone) or "E" (estrogen) have no idea what is in store for them if they stay on that regimen. If they were informed that the consequences of cross-sex hormones may include "excruciating genital growth, vaginal atrophy and tearing, and much higher risk for cancer and cardiovascular disease," would they readily assent?[208] And are fourteen- or fifteen-year-olds even capable of giving such assent?

Despite the happy talk found on trans websites, hormone therapy is less a bed of roses than a bed of nails. Physiotherapist Elaine Miller told *The Telegraph* of London that women on testosterone were achieving the equivalent of menopause twenty to thirty years ahead of schedule. Mood swings are the least of it. Said Miller: "Wetting yourself is something that just is not socially acceptable, and it stops people from exercising, it stops them from having intimate relationships, it stops them from travelling, it has work impacts."[209]

I ask again: Is a fourteen-year-old girl capable of making this sort of profoundly life-altering decision?

In some cases, the effects of sex hormones will fade if one ceases usage. This depends upon dose, duration, and the individual. Certain detransitioners have actually resumed normal reproductive function and become pregnant. So infertility is not a given, but it is a strong possibility. We just don't know—and trans advocates have little interest in finding the answers to these questions.

---

[207] Lyvia Maria Bezerra da Silva et al., "Pelvic Floor Dysfunction in Transgender Men on Gender-affirming Hormone Therapy: A Descriptive Cross-sectional Study," *International Urogynecology Journal* 35 (2024): 1077–1084.

[208] Sapir, "The reckoning over puberty blockers has arrived."

[209] Eliza Mondegreen, "The hidden long-term risks of youth gender transition," UnHerd, May 28, 2024.

A full accounting of the health risks associated with cross-sex hormones would stretch on for many pages, but the highly respected Washington, DC, law firm Cooper & Kirk, in a white paper prepared for Do No Harm, summarizes them as such:

> For males, the use of cross-sex hormones is associated with numerous health risks, such as thromboembolic disease, including blood clots; cholelithiasis, including gallstones; coronary artery disease, including heart attacks; macroprolactinoma, which is a tumor of the pituitary gland; cerebrovascular disease, including strokes; hypertriglyceridemia, which is an elevated level of triglycerides in the blood; breast cancer; and irreversible infertility. For females, the use of cross-sex hormones is associated with risks of erythrocytosis, which is an increase in red blood cells; severe liver dysfunction; coronary artery disease, including heart attacks; depression; hypertension; infertility; and increased risk of breast, cervical, and uterine cancers.[210]

Surgery is the final step in the transition from male or female to… well, to an altered form of male or female. Patients change their physical characteristics but it is preposterous to claim that they change their sex. Males who take estrogen will never have normal development of their penis, and women on high doses of testosterone will have abnormal vaginal epitheliums, but they're not really changing their sex. They're also at risk for fistulas, the need for a colostomy, loss of sexual sensation, and a variety of equally unpleasant conditions.

"Gender-affirming surgery" is cosmetic surgery. No matter the insistence upon transposed (or made-up) pronouns, men who take estrogen

---

210 Cooper & Kirk, PLLC, David H. Thompson, Brian W. Barnes, and John D. Ramer, "The Justice for Adolescent and Child Transitioners Act (The JUST FACTS Act)," Do No Harm, January 2023.

or have their penises removed may look different but they are not women, just as people who take Botox injections may look younger but they are not really younger.

Girls who don't want to have periods will have their uteruses removed, their ovaries taken out. Boys may have their testicles and penis excised. Pseudo vaginas and artificial penises may be attached via metoidioplasties and penectomies, but they can't produce eggs or sperm, and the X-Y or X-X chromosomes remain.

So "sex reassignment surgery" is as speciously false a phrase as "age-repealing Botox therapy." Patients change their appearance, not their sex or their age.

In 2004, Paul R. McHugh, University Distinguished Service Professor of Psychiatry at Johns Hopkins University, published a moving essay in *First Things* about why Hopkins, under his leadership, stopped doing surgical sex procedures for adults with gender dysphoria. Though his focus was on adults and ours at Do No Harm is strictly on minors, Dr. McHugh explained the seeming impossibility of a switch from male to female. (Recall that in the late twentieth and early twenty-first centuries, before the explosion of late-onset gender dysphoria in teenaged girls, the overwhelming majority of transitions were male to female.)

"The post-surgical subjects struck me as caricatures of women," said Dr. McHugh. "They wore high heels, copious makeup, and flamboyant clothing; they spoke about how they found themselves able to give vent to their natural inclinations for peace, domesticity, and gentleness—but their large hands, prominent Adam's apples, and thick facial features were incongruous (and would become more so as they aged). Women psychiatrists whom I sent to talk with them would intuitively see through the disguise and the exaggerated postures. 'Gals know gals,' one said to me, 'and that's a guy.'"[211]

Surely this is heartbreaking for the subjects of such surgery, but they are adults and have the right to undergo the procedure. To believe

---

[211]   Paul R. McHugh, "Surgical Sex," *First Things*, November 2004.

that minors are capable of so momentous and irreversible a decision is preposterous.

(Trans men have a more difficult time changing appearance, which is the root of the "misgendering" contretemps that pop up on social media from time to time. I have a high-pitched voice and once or twice a stranger has addressed me as "Ma'am" over the phone, but this was hardly cause for throwing a hissy fit.)

After recounting the lacerated vaginas, enlarged clitorises, and microphalluses of the young people who emerged from the Washington University of St. Louis Transgender Center, Jamie Reed, a courageous whistleblower, concluded, "There are rare conditions in which babies are born with atypical genitalia—cases that call for sophisticated care and compassion. But clinics like the one where I worked are *creating* a whole cohort of kids with atypical genitals—and most of these teens haven't even had sex yet. They had no idea who they were going to be as adults. Yet all it took for them to permanently transform themselves was one or two short conversations with a therapist."[212]

- - - - - -

Many Americans today who fill out forms before seeing their doctor are given a box to check that asks for "Sex Assigned at Birth"—as if inditing M or F on a birth certificate is a mere matter of whim!

That so risibly absurd a phrase has penetrated so far into the bureaucratic paper-pushing world would be funny if it weren't so dispiriting. I guess the ob-gyn, upon delivering a baby, flips a coin and arbitrarily "assigns" the baby to Team Boy or Team Girl. The clearly visible sex organs play at most a supporting role in this capricious decision.

Incredibly, medical schools teach this twaddle. Anatomy courses instruct medical students that sex is a spectrum. The rationale is that

---

[212] Jamie Reed, "I Thought I Was Saving Trans Kids. Now I'm Blowing the Whistle," *The Free Press*, February 9, 2023, https://www.thefp.com/p/i-thought-i-was-saving-trans-kids.

some tiny number of unfortunate people are born with abnormally developed sex organs. The thing is, this is not a spectrum; it's an abnormality. There are people born with congenital heart disease. That doesn't mean there is a spectrum of what a heart should be like. There's a normal heart and various abnormal hearts.

Medical schools commit intellectual malpractice by teaching medical students that a person can be any sex he or she wishes to be.

Endocrinologist Roy Eappen, a Do No Harm senior fellow, and others have argued that at its base, the trans movement is an attempt to erase gay people. It's called "transing away the gay."

Current thinking has it that being gay has a deep and strong biological basis. The now discredited practice of trying to convince gay people that they can "convert" to heterosexuality was known as conversion therapy. Yet to take gay people and try to convince them that they are not gay but rather were born in the wrong sex is an even more extreme form of conversion therapy.[213]

We know, from voluminous evidence, that there is an extremely high likelihood that childhood-onset gender incongruence will resolve on its own by adolescence or adulthood. That this resolution will not infrequently be in the form of a gay or lesbian identity explains why many gay people view the trans phenomenon as anti-gay. For instance, there are only thirty-two lesbian bars left in America. There are various reasons cited for this, among them increased acceptance of gay people in public spaces and the explosion of online dating, but it's hard not to think that the trans war on gayness hasn't something to do with it.[214]

---

[213] One heterosexually oriented trans cohort consists of men who have autogynephilia, which is a condition in which one is sexually aroused by imagining or seeing himself dressed as a woman. Paul R. McHugh, the distinguished psychiatrist at Johns Hopkins, writes that transgender activists have lodged "protests against the diagnosis of autogynephilia as a mechanism to generate demands for sex-change operations, but they have offered little evidence to refute the diagnosis." Paul R. McHugh, "Surgical Sex."

[214] Alani Vargas, "'Lesbian Bars Near Me': Where the 32 Remaining Lesbian Bars Are in America," *Parade*, updated April 23, 2024.

There have been cross-dressers, transvestites, and those who adopt a persona of the other sex for as long as humans have donned clothes. This will never disappear and we have no reason to wish it to do so. Do No Harm is only concerned when minors are involved.

Sadly, we are witnessing the abolition of the venerable and very charming category of the "tomboy," defined as "a girl who enjoys rough, noisy activities traditionally associated with boys."[215] In the past, such behavior was seen as perfectly normal. In fact, most tomboys grew into heterosexual women. Today, a disturbingly large number of tomboys would be pushed down the trans highway by the pressure of peers, popular culture, social media, and trans activists.

As for the pronouns business, part of a physician's job is to make the patient feel comfortable and have trust in us. If a patient wants to be called by a name other than his or her birth name, even one traditionally bestowed upon the opposite sex—Caitlyn, Ralph, Napoleon, whatever—I will call him or her by that name. Patients have special privileges, and I have no desire to antagonize them, as antagonized patients are impossible to deal with. But I'm not going to call anyone by a pronoun at odds with their sex, any more than I will say that two plus two equals five. That's nonsense, and I will not be coerced or bullied into participating in farce.

I'll call you whatever you want to be called. But don't tell me I'm going to lose my job if I misspeak or fail to use one of the crazy pronouns—zir and the like—that virtue-signalers prize. That's ridiculous, and you have no right to force anyone else to appear ridiculous.

The trump card of the trans movement is the ominous threat of teen suicide. When a parent is told that a child will quite probably take his or her own life if not encouraged or at least permitted to transition,

---

[215] Oxford Languages, https://languages.oup.com/google-dictionary-en.

that parent will frequently accede to whatever is demanded. After all, no specter haunts a parent more than a child's death.

As the Washington University of St. Louis Transgender Center's website warns, "Left untreated, gender dysphoria has any number of consequences, from self-harm to suicide. But when you take away the gender dysphoria by allowing a child to be who he or she is, we're noticing that goes away. The studies we have show these kids often wind up functioning psychosocially as well as or better than their peers."[216]

This specter is a mendacious mirage. Yes, the rate of suicide in gender-confused children is comparatively high, but it is no higher than for children suffering other psychiatric problems. When people are in turmoil, they are likelier to commit self-harm. But there is no evidence that "gender-affirming care" lessens this danger. To assert otherwise is to engage in shameless coercion.

Yet the by now clichéd claim that 41 percent of trans-identifying people attempt suicide is a specious untruth that has somehow gained the status of conventional wisdom. It has also given rise to a particularly loathsome form of blackmail, as parents who are not supportive of a child's desire to transition are asked if they'd rather have "a live son or a dead daughter" or vice versa.

The 41 percent figure comes from "Suicide Attempts among Transgender and Gender Non-Conforming Adults: Findings of The National Transgender Discrimination Survey," a 2014 report by researchers from the American Foundation for Suicide Prevention and the Williams Institute at the UCLA School of Law.

The 2008 survey upon which the report was based, which included more than six thousand respondents, did indeed record an attempted suicide rate of 41 percent for transgender-identifying people, which is about ten times the rate of the general population and more than twice the rate of gays and lesbians. This is a disturbingly, tragically high

---

[216] Reed, "I Thought I Was Saving Trans Kids. Now I'm Blowing the Whistle."

number, but as the authors themselves point out, the survey was hamstrung by several serious limitations.

For one thing, the questionnaire asked only one question about suicidal behavior: "Have you ever attempted suicide?" The only answers were yes and no. The authors note, "Researchers have found that using this question alone in surveys can inflate the percentage of affirmative responses, since some respondents may use it to communicate self-harm behavior that is not a 'suicide attempt,' such as seriously considering suicide, planning for suicide, or engaging in self-harm behavior without the intent to die." In another study, deeper probing about the intent to commit suicide resulted in a greater than 40 percent reduction of reported attempted suicides in the general population, from 4.6 percent to 2.7 percent.

Moreover, the survey did not attempt to ascertain the mental health status or the history of traumatic events among respondents—both important risk factors in suicide ideation and attempts. Interestingly, "respondents who said they had received transition-related health care or wanted to have it someday were more likely to report having attempted suicide than those who said they did not want it."[217] This raises but does not answer the question of whether medical transitioning decreases—or increases—the likelihood of a suicide attempt.

Reporting on Suicide, a compilation of best practices and recommendations gathered in consultation from more than two dozen international organizations and nonprofits dealing with self-harm, includes among its recommendations two injunctions regularly violated by the gender-transition complex:

---

[217] Ann P. Haas, Philip L. Rodgers, and Jody L. Herman, "Suicide Attempts among Transgender and Gender Non-Conforming Adults: Findings of The National Transgender Discrimination Survey," American Foundation for Suicide Prevention and the Williams Institute, January 2014.

— "Provide context and facts to counter perceptions that the suicide was tied to heroism, honor, or loyalty to an individual or group."

— Do not "[o]verstat[e] the problem of suicide by using descriptors like 'epidemic' or 'skyrocketing.'"[218]

Alas, treating the suicide issue more honestly and retiring the 41 percent statistic is not in the trans industry's self-interest—and at latest report, that industry's self-interest is immense…and rising.

— — — — — —

The anti-child transitioning movement is passionate, cogent, and growing by the day. It comprises a diverse coalition of physicians, medical experts, concerned citizens, detransitioners, and mothers whose children have gone through this. This last-named group is strong, outspoken, and deeply committed.

Writing for 4thWaveNow, which calls itself "a community of people who question the medicalization of gender-atypical youth," Marie Verite and Brie J (critical thinkers who write on this subject often use pseudonyms due to the viciousness of some trans activists toward perceived "turncoats") say they "find it mystifying that a preference for desistance is even controversial. Surely, if a child can find peace in his or her unaltered body—and happily avoid becoming a sterilized medical patient dependent for life on drugs and surgeries—that is a positive outcome."[219]

4thWaveNow consists largely of parents who support their children's "gender discordance" while casting a skeptical eye on the idea that this translates to "bodily discordance." Interestingly, a good number of the anti-child trans crowd are pro-LGBT and supporters of gay marriage. But they believe that encouraging children to mutilate their bodies

---

[218] "Best Practices and Recommendations for Reporting on Suicide," Reporting on Suicide, https://reportingonsuicide.org/recommendations/.

[219] Marie Verite and Brie J, "'Intellectual no-platforming': Ken Zucker pushes back on the latest attempt to discredit desistance-persistence research," 4thWaveNow, May 30, 2018.

rather than accept same-sex attraction is profoundly anti-gay. And they are correct. You don't need to radically alter your body and become a lifelong patient of the medical-pharmaceutical complex in order to marry the adult of your choice. After all, it is by now well-established that most—anywhere from two-thirds to 98 percent—of prepubertal gender dysphoric children will desist by the time they hit adolescence.[220] And most of these children will grow into gay or lesbian adults.

The writers at 4thWaveNow ask if it wouldn't be "more compassionate and prudent" to help gender-confused girls "accept themselves as females who simply don't fit societal gender norms? Many of these girls, prior to transition, live a lesbian lifestyle (even if they reject the label 'lesbian'). How much kinder would it be to help them embrace the only bodies they will ever have, with the sexual preference they have, instead of endorsing extreme interventions **that may never resolve their dysphoria?** [bold in original]"[221]

We don't have good numbers on the percentage of young people who step off the trans train at its various junctions before surgery. A not insignificant number of individuals drop out of this life, but we've really no idea how many they are, and we probably won't have a good idea for another five to ten years, since this trend began taking shape in 2009 and accelerated about 2014.

One study suggests that perhaps 30 percent of those on hormone therapy stop taking the medication, but many do not wish to come forward and admit to the terrible mistake they have made.[222]

Those researching the subject are almost uniformly pro-trans activists and thus about as trustworthy as your typical propagandist. They will never come to a conclusion contrary to their own prejudices. So we

---

220   Leor Sapir, "The School-to-Clinic Pipeline," *City Journal*, Autumn 2022.
221   "The 41% trans suicide attempt rate: A tale of flawed data and lazy journalists," 4thWaveNow, August 3, 2015.
222   Pranav Gupta et al., "Continuation of Gender-Affirming Hormone Therapy in Transgender and Gender-Diverse Individuals: A Systematic Review," *Endocrine Practice* 30, no. 12 (December 2024): 1206–1211, https://pubmed.ncbi.nlm.nih.gov/39306093.

simply do not have an objective, dispassionate accounting of the detransitioning experience.

As with so much in this puzzling field, we just don't know who drops out or why. When does the regret kick in: after five years, ten years, and for some people, never? It's all guesswork at this point.

That doesn't stop the more fanatical gender clinicians from downplaying the potential complications. Dr. Johanna Olson-Kennedy, an adolescent medicine physician and medical director at the Center for Transyouth Health and Development at Children's Hospital of Los Angeles, has even pooh-poohed the magnitude of a young woman's choice to undergo voluntary mastectomy. She says, "If you want breasts at a later point in your life, you can go and get them."[223]

This is a remarkably cavalier treatment of a momentous decision in one's life, but gender activists say the same thing about the loss of fertility. "If you want a child later in life, you can always adopt." True, but is this an irrevocable choice one should make at age fifteen? Might not a woman feel differently about this at age twenty-five than she did a decade earlier?

Or what of the disproportionate number of trans patients who are autistic, depressed, schizophrenic, or abused? They are not thinking rationally. Their lives have been a disaster. Must they go through this potentially traumatic "journey" in order to satisfy the ideologues?

Not all damage can be repaired. A uterine transplant is theoretically possible—a penis transplant less so—but so much of this is redolent of *Frankenstein*.

Dr. Olson-Kennedy ought to speak to Chloe Cole, a young woman who is among Do No Harm's most eloquent spokespeople. Chloe is a bright and lovely young woman who has been evaluated as a highly functioning autistic. Severely depressed, she began social transformation at the age of twelve. She soon moved into puberty blockers followed by sex hormones, and at the criminally early age of fifteen she underwent a

---

[223] Mondegreen, "The hidden long-term risks of youth gender transition."

double mastectomy in which her breasts were removed and her nipples were grafted.

At sixteen, Chloe had a revelation. Or maybe it was just maturation. Her gender confusion cleared. She was interested in boys. She hopped off the trans train—but she's left with no breasts, weeping incisions, and gynecological problems that are probably the result of exposure to high levels of testosterone.

She testified in 2022 before the Florida Boards of Medicine and Osteopathic Medicine Joint Rules/Legislative Committee, "I want to be a mother someday, and yet I can never naturally feed…my future children. My breasts were beautiful and now they have been incinerated for nothing. Thank you, modern medicine."[224]

In 2024, Chloe presented the annual shareholders' meeting of Disney with a Do No Harm proposal to correct an inequity in its employee benefits package. The company, she pointed out to its shareholders, "pays for gender transition interventions, but not detransitioning care. Therefore, the Company discriminates based on gender identity, under EEOC regulations."

Chloe laid out her backstory:

> Influenced by modern media and social networks, I began a transition to male at age 12. By age 16, after practitioners I trusted encouraged me to take puberty blockers and get a double mastectomy, I tried to come back to reality. But it was too late.
>
> My body has been irreversibly damaged, and years later, my chest is still in bandages. My doctors have abandoned me. New doctors look and shrug. As a result, I am suing those professionals who steered me into

---

[224] Joseph MacKinnon, "De-transitioner warns shareholders that Disney will pay a price for 'stealing the voices of thousands of little Ariels,'" Blaze Media, April 5, 2024.

taking these destructive steps that have permanently scarred me.

Disney rejected her proposal, but Chloe left CEO Bob Iger with a warning: "The lawsuits are coming, sir. It's only a matter of time before current or past employees, whose bodies and lives have been irreversibly harmed, will show up at your door looking for justice and restitution."[225]

This brave and indefatigable young woman is already at the door of Kaiser Permanente, seeking justice and restitution. Chloe's is among the fifty or so lawsuits that are planned or have been filed against those who in various ways have encouraged or effected the transition of minors.

Dr. Paul McHugh of Johns Hopkins predicts that a flood of lawsuits will come when girls who have undergone gender-altering treatment "wake up at age twenty-three, twenty-four, and say, 'Here I am. I've got a five-o'clock shadow, I'm mutilated and I'm sterile, and I'm not what I ought to be. How did this happen?'"[226]

What about the tougher cases in which a parent consents to radical treatment?

There is an analogue, at least tangentially, to Christian Scientist parents who have refused blood transfusions or other necessary treatments for their sick children. Obviously parents must be involved in their children's medical care. But do they have the right to choose care that will worsen their children's condition?

What are the limits of parental control over a child's well-being? At what point may the state step in to protect the child? I concede that this is a complicated, murky philosophical issue.

The question turns on informed consent. Were the nature and consequences of puberty blockers, hormone treatments, and surgery properly explained to the young transitioners? Were they coerced into these

---

[225] Heather Hunter, "Detransitioner Chloe Cole warns Disney CEO Bob Iger that 'lawsuits are coming,'" *Washington Examiner*, April 3, 2024.

[226] Shrier, *Irreversible Damage: The Transgender Craze Seducing Our Daughters*, 142.

treatments? Were they told the whole truth about the treatments they were about to undergo?

If these lawsuits work, childhood gender transition will cease. Medical institutions, pharmaceutical companies, and physicians will not expose themselves to potentially astronomical judgments. (Professional societies that put out standards of care are also the targets of some suits, as they should be.) A small number of adults will continue to opt for medical and surgical treatments. These will continue. But not for children.

— — — — — —

The most important study forwarded by those who believe transitioning improves the psychological well-being of children came out of the University of Washington. The subjects, ages thirteen to twenty, identified as trans, nonbinary, or "I don't know" and were seeking care at Seattle Children's Hospital's Gender Clinic. Their mean age was 15.8 years.

At the end of twelve months—a scandalously short interval—the UW team looked at the psychological profiles of the two groups. Those who had received "gender-affirming" treatment were said to have had lower odds of depression and suicidality. This is somewhat misleading: in fact, their rates of depression and suicidality before and after treatment saw no statistically significant change, but the psychological health of those who did not receive puberty blockers and/or hormones declined.[227]

On its face, this seemed significant. But the study had a serious, even disabling, problem. Heroic journalist Jesse Singal, who debunked the study, explains:

> [A]ny genuine comparison between the GAM [gen-der-affirming medicine] and no-GAM kids 12 months

---

227   Diana M. Tordoff et al., "Mental Health Outcomes in Transgender and Nonbinary Youths Receiving Gender-Affirming Care," *JAMA Network Open* 5, no. 2 (February 2022).

out is impossible, because 80% of the kids who didn't go on GAM had dropped out of the study by the final wave of data collection, leaving just six remaining. That is far too small a sample to draw any conclusions from.[228]

We have no idea if the kids who left the study were now satisfied with their gender, still depressed and suicidal, or what. Yet this finding is cited in nearly every review of the subject as evidence of the benefits of transformation. This is an awfully wobbly plank upon which to base the case for putting someone on medications for the rest of his or her life, cutting off breasts and penises, and otherwise altering the lives of confused boys and girls.

Another well-publicized study, this one appearing in the once-august pages of the *New England Journal of Medicine*, claimed that juveniles taking sex-characteristic-altering hormones experienced increased satisfaction with their physical appearance and improved psychosocial functioning.[229]

If this had been an unbiased study by scholars without any axes to grind it would have been interesting. Unfortunately, the researchers and four clinics featured in this study had well-publicized histories of radical activism and advocacy for the medical transition of children. For example, Boston Children's Hospital posted and later removed a video on its YouTube channel that endorsed the idea that some children know their gender identity "from the womb." The University of California, San Francisco website endorses the idea that naturopathic providers are well-suited to prescribe gender-affirming hormones. Lurie Children's Hospital of Chicago has disseminated "educational" materials to local schools that recommend that schools "automatically 'affirm' students who announce sexual transitions, and 'communicate a non-binary

---

[228] Jesse Singal, "The University of Washington Is Putting Trans Kids At Risk By Distorting Suicide Research," *Singal-Minded*, September 21, 2022, https://jessesingal.substack.com/p/the-university-of-washington-is-putting.

[229] Diane Chen et al., "Psychosocial Functioning in Transgender Youth after 2 Years of Hormones," *New England Journal of Medicine* 388, no. 3 (2023): 240–250.

understanding of gender' to children in the classrooms…to disrupt the 'entrenched [gender] norms in western society.'"[230] One coauthor of the paper is the notorious Johanna Olson-Kennedy, she of the infamous "If you want breasts at a later point in your life, you can go and get them" quote.

Given the obvious and even outrageous bias of the authors, there is a high probability that study participants were steered toward responses that align with the activism promoted by these clinics. This phenomenon—known as "demand characteristics"—is a remarkably well-documented threat to the validity of survey-based scientific inquiry, even for researchers who do their best to conduct studies dispassionately and objectively.

The study suffers from other major flaws as well. Its results indicate that the only meaningful improvement over time was participant scores for "appearance congruence." Life satisfaction, depression, and anxiety only improved by the smallest margins. Notably, the study does not include comparison groups that received psychotherapy or no intervention at all, so whether these modest improvements are superior to alternative approaches is impossible to assess.

The researchers observed extremely modest self-reported mental health improvement among participants who began taking gender-affirming hormones later in puberty, but static measures among those who started taking these hormones early in puberty. They explain that "these observations align with other published reports that earlier access to gender affirming medical care is associated with more positive psychosocial functioning." In other words, they claim that the lack of improvement within this subsample constitutes evidence in support of their radical worldview. It's a "heads I win, tails you lose" proposition.

This study, like others by ideologically motivated authors, obfuscates rather than clarifies questions around the medical transition of children. Citizens and policymakers must accept the unfortunate fact

---

[230]   Christopher F. Rufo, "Unholy Alliance," *City Journal*, August 31, 2022.

that elite gatekeepers have become cheerleaders for transitioning; their recommendations on politicized topics warrant healthy skepticism.

With greater clarity, a group of scholars undertook a study of the quality of life of fifty-five transsexuals (all but three were male to female) who had received hormonal treatments at the University Hospital of Bern in Switzerland. The subjects of the study had transitioned at least fifteen years earlier. Compared to a control group of healthy female medical staff who had undergone at least one pelvic or abdominal operation, the transsexuals expressed "significantly lower" satisfaction with their general health and personal, physical, and role limitations. (The transsexuals and the members of the control group expressed similar levels of satisfaction with emotions, sleep, and incontinence.)[231]

This is consistent with previous and non-politicized research. In 2004, *The Guardian* retained the Aggressive Research Intelligence Facility (ARIF) of the University of Birmingham to conduct a review of over "100 international medical studies of post-operative transsexuals."

ARIF found "no robust scientific evidence that gender reassignment surgery is effective," reported the newspaper. As with the previously mentioned University of Washington study, many of the ostensibly scientific investigations assessed by ARIF were marred by enormous dropout rates. In one case, 495 of the 727 post-operative transsexuals left the five-year study.

The ARIF scholars noted that the poorly designed research projects often "skewed the results to suggest that sex change operations are beneficial"—and this was more than two decades ago, before the teen-girl gender-dysphoria craze and the egregious politicization of the trans-industrial complex.

---

[231] Annette Kuhn et al., "Quality of life 15 years after sex reassignment surgery for transsexualism," *Fertility and Sterility* 92, no. 5 (November 2009). There is a parallel question here of whether self-reported satisfaction with a medical procedure has any connection with "objective measurements of mental health and psychosocial functioning." See Leor Sapir, "A Slow Trek Back to Truth?" *City Journal*, August 25, 2023.

Dr. Chris Hyde, director of ARIF, told *The Guardian* that "a large number of people who have the surgery…remain traumatized—often to the point of committing suicide." He concluded, "The bottom line is that although it's clear that some people do well with gender reassignment surgery, the available research does little to reassure about how many patients do badly and, if so, how badly."[232]

To gamble the lives of confused children and teenagers on such a risky life-and-death proposition is unworthy of a decent society.

---

[232] David Batty, "Sex changes are not effective, say researchers," *The Guardian*, July 30, 2004.

CHAPTER SEVEN

TURNING THE TRANS TIDE

Sometimes, all it takes is one courageous and enlightened person to reverse a disastrous tide—whether it's the little boy who notices and calls out that the emperor has no clothes or it's a brave clinician, a gutsy whistleblower, a truth-seeking journalist, or an influential intellectual who sees the madness and says, "Enough!"

At the time of her whistleblowing in 2023, Jamie Reed described herself as a "42-year-old St. Louis native, a queer woman, and to the left of Bernie Sanders," and married to a transgender man. So she is not the intolerant Bible-thumping "transphobe" of common caricature. Yet she courageously blew the whistle on the Washington University Transgender Center at St. Louis Children's Hospital.

From 2018 to 2022, Reed was a case manager at the Wash U Transgender Center. She was responsible for intake and oversight of the nearly one thousand "distressed young people" who had come through its doors. Her story, which she detailed in an extraordinary essay that was published in February 2023 in the *Free Press*, provided a shocking look inside the trans industry.

Jamie witnessed firsthand the sea change in trans patients, as the traditional profile—a very young boy who wanted to be a girl—was swamped in number by teenaged girls with no previous history of gender dysphoria but who "suddenly declared they were transgender and demanded immediate treatment with testosterone." These girls had numerous comorbidities—anxiety, depression, anorexia, obesity, autism—as well as "false self-diagnoses" such as multiple personalities. She also saw a disturbing number of girls who had been referred from the inpatient psychiatric unit of the St. Louis Children's Hospital—kids who had been diagnosed with bipolar disorder, schizophrenia, and other mental illnesses.

Jamie was appalled by the way the clinic hustled kids through transitions. She raised the possibility that clusters of transition-seeking girls from the same school could be a sign of social contagion, but her superiors dismissed this concern. All a patient needed to be placed on the path to transition was a letter from one therapist—"usually one we recommended." The Transgender Center supplied a template for such a letter. An endocrinologist then wrote a prescription for testosterone, and the die was cast.

"I came to believe," said Jamie Reed, "that teenagers are simply not capable of fully grasping what it means to make the decision to become infertile while still a minor."

Although Jamie had received sterling performance reviews over the years, her reluctance to participate in an assembly-line process that hurried confused people on a road from which there is no full return attracted the attention of her superiors. She was told to accept "medicine and the science" and "Get on board, or get out." Her sins included raising objections to bypassing parents in transition decisions. As she insisted in a January 2022 email to a staff therapist, "I do not ethically agree with linking a minor patient to a therapist who would be gender affirming with gender as a focus of their work without that being discussed with the parents and the parent agreeing to that kind of care."

You might think that Jamie's position was unassailable. Parents should have a say in whether their minor child is being encouraged by medical authorities to undergo a gender transition. But this industry is so far gone in trans-for-kids mania that hers was a controversial statement.

In November 2022, Jamie left the Wash U Transgender Center for another job with the Washington University School of Medicine, this one coordinating studies of children receiving bone marrow transplants. But she couldn't unsee what she had seen, and she couldn't remain silent. The trigger came when she read an article stating that Dr. Rachel Levine, assistant secretary for health in the US Department of Health and Human Services, "said that clinics are proceeding carefully and that no American children are receiving drugs or hormones for gender dysphoria who shouldn't."

So she blew the whistle on the Transgender Center. Jamie bravely wrote a lengthy piece for the *Free Press* and brought her concerns to the attorney general of the state of Missouri. "He is a Republican," she said, and "I am a progressive. But the safety of children should not be a matter for our culture wars."[233]

The corporate and mainstream media act as cheerleaders or at least stenographers for the trans-industrial complex. On the infrequent occasions that a reporter introduces a note of skepticism or evenhandedness, the complex goes into full censorship mode. So when the *New York Times* ran a balanced story about Jamie Reed and the Wash U clinic, GLAAD, a pressure group that seeks to ensure one-sidedly favorable coverage of LGBTQ—especially TQ—issues, "parked a van outside the *NYT*'s offices, emblazoned in block capitals with the demand: 'Stop questioning trans people's right to exist & access medical care.'"

The group went on to call Jamie Reed's claims "debunked lies from an anti-trans extremist." As Josephine Bartosch of UnHerd noted, the GLAAD hysterics obviously did not read the article, which made clear

---

233   Reed, "I Thought I Was Saving Trans Kids. Now I'm Blowing the Whistle."

that Jamie Reed is a lesbian with a trans partner.[234] Listening, like taking the time to understand the position of those who disagree with them, is not a strength of the trans industry.

The vituperation directed at Jamie Reed was not out of character for trans activists. You know the world has turned upside down when Chase Strangio, the deputy director for transgender justice at the American Civil Liberties Union—the ACLU!—tweets about Abigail Shrier's best-seller, *Irreversible Damage: The Transgender Craze Seducing Our Daughters*, "Stopping the circulation of this book and these ideas is 100% a hill I will die on."[235] I'm afraid Strangio took the ACLU's integrity with him.

As in other realms of medicine, practitioners of identity politics thrive on vengeance and wield the pink slip as a primary weapon.

Beth Rempe, a nurse on the Do No Harm team, confronted the unpleasant reality that our medical institutions have been saturated with woke ideology. With courage and conviction, she stood up and said no—and was forced out for sticking to her principles.

Beth was a full-time nurse at Georgetown University Hospital and Children's National Medical Center in Washington, DC, who took a part-time role in the gastrointestinal unit at Children's. She was well-respected and had earned seniority of schedule. Beth loved her job, and the staff and patients at Children's loved her back.

Then came her crucible.

Beth's team started being assigned regular training modules on LGBTQ+ issues, with one video that lasted two hours, far more than they had experienced in the past. This specific video focused on gender ideology and transition for children, utilizing a gender unicorn as an example of how to assess young children.

---

[234] Josephine Bartosch, "The *New York Times* is finally standing up to trans censorship," UnHerd, August 25, 2023.
[235] Shrier, *Irreversible Damage: The Transgender Craze Seducing Our Daughters*, xix.

This escalated into regular ongoing training that was not focused on medical procedures and new treatments, but instead on how to use correct pronouns and showcase one's inclusivity. The regimen included a lengthy session on microaggressions.

Beth sensed a bad moon rising. She worried that soon she would be forced to treat children undergoing gender transitions and provide them with treatments with which she profoundly disagreed.

Beth went to her supervisor with her concerns. She was told that her work was greatly appreciated and assured that she had nothing to worry about.

In 2021, Beth was assigned her first young patient who identified as transgender. She told her supervisor that she was morally opposed to and would be unable to administer treatments that would be part of the transition.

Beth explains:

> When I approached my supervisor about asking for an exemption from participating in gender-affirming care, I made it clear that I would treat the patient with absolute care and respect as I administered any other necessary care that the patient needed. I just couldn't do anything that promoted gender transition.

Her supervisor lacked the authority to grant an exemption, so together the two of them brought Beth's request to the nursing director of acute care, who in turn brought it to the hospital administration, which consulted with the American Nurses Association. Administrators informed her that she would not receive an exemption from participation and that she had to use the patient's preferred pronouns and name, but due to Beth's standing at the hospital and their eagerness to keep her on the team, they encouraged her to stay, hoping that she would not encounter any kindred situations.

But she did. The next twelve months brought a rapid influx of teenage girls identifying as transgender. These children overwhelmingly had coexisting mental issues and had suffered sexual abuse and other traumas.

Beth's eyes were opened.

"Watching how every member of the medical teams 100% affirmed the male identity of the troubled teen girls admitted to my unit was sad and shocking. It would be obvious to anyone that these girls had much more going on that led them to choose this identity."

At one point, the twelve-bed unit had one or two transitioning young patients at all times. There was no way Beth could avoid the issue.

The hospital didn't fire Beth. In fact, her supervisors expressed how much they valued her on numerous occasions. But her deep convictions that these treatments were wrong—and the way the medical staff encouraged children to pursue gender transition—forced upon Beth a difficult choice.

To avoid putting her supervisor in the awkward position of firing her, Beth resigned. The nursing profession lost a bright, passionate, caring professional, all because she would not participate in what she regarded as cruel, inhumane treatment of confused young people.

Today, Beth reflects:

> It was sad for me to consider how many very skilled and caring healthcare professionals had to go along with the gender ideology just to continue practicing at Children's. To those experiencing this, you are not alone. It may seem like everyone you work with is following an ideology that is destructive. Remember that there are many people outside of your institution that agree with you.

This is a case of ideology driving medical care. It's the opposite of inclusion, for you can only be included if you pledge allegiance (even if cynically) to the party line.

We don't have this problem in other areas of medicine. We don't have nurses say, "I don't like dialysis." And if someone did say this, we'd ask him or her why and come to an understanding. But there is no understanding—no good faith—no live and let live—when it comes to trans matters. Dissenters are libeled as transphobes and instructed to get the hell out.

Stephanie Winn, a licensed marriage and family therapist in Oregon, also fell afoul of the punishment-minded.

Stephanie, who had worked with patients with gender identity problems, noticed that their comorbidities—histories of sexual trauma, autistic traits, or compulsive disorders—were not being addressed. "Some were homosexual and hadn't seemed to grapple with that, or hadn't had sexual experiences or relationships yet," she says. Others seemed to be using gender identity as a form of teenage rebellion, or a weapon in family conflict. Their problems did not go away after ostensibly switching sexes.

Stephanie's eyes were opened further when she learned of detransitioners. "They were not mentioned, as far as I can recall, in the training. And just the idea that anybody ever regretted this had never come up."

When Stephanie shared the experiences of detransitioners on her blog and podcast, "You Must Be Some Kind of Therapist," trans activists fell into their all-too-common pattern of waging personal and professional attacks on her. They accused her of conversion therapy, a charge which could have resulted in the loss of her license. She was rightfully cleared of all charges with no disciplinary action, and she refused to be intimidated. Stephanie continues to provide patients and parents with the best possible care, though she has stopped working with minors who identify as transgender.

Stephanie believes that helping detransitioners heal is essential to restoring integrity to the profession of psychotherapy. "Detransitioners have the most reason out of anybody to mistrust therapists because many of them have been permanently physically harmed," she says. Many feel a sense of rage toward the doctors, therapists, and others who pushed them toward their decisions.

She does not spare her fellow therapists from blame. Many of Stephanie's colleagues have the "attitude that if I'm being told something by an expert in the field that seems counterintuitive or strange to me, it must be because they know something I don't know." So these kids get a pass-through from therapists—and are pushed down a road they will likely regret having taken.

While the US healthcare establishment has been captured by the most radical elements of the trans movement—those which advocate chemical and surgical mutilation of children—Northern and Western Europe, which exhibit US-like levels of support for transgenderism among adults, are rejecting "gender-affirming care" for children.

Several countries, including the United Kingdom, Sweden, and Finland, have explicitly abandoned "gender affirmation" in recent years in part due to fear that medical intervention has become overprescribed. They are fully aware—as somehow many American medical establishments are not—that studies show that only a small number of cases of childhood gender dysphoria persist into adulthood.[236]

The practical reality is that transgender treatments for minors are increasingly off-limits in Europe, with some countries effectively ending them in all but rare cases or outside rigorously controlled clinical trials. Yet many states in America raise few if any barriers, even to younger children. It is striking that countries generally regarded as the most sexually progressive in the Western world, such as Sweden, are notably more conservative in safeguarding children than is the United States.

In a sharp departure from the gender-affirmation model employed in the United States, which is now regrettably the most permissive country

---

[236] "Reassigned," Do No Harm, January 16, 2023.

in the world when it comes to the legal and medical gender transition of minors, these European nations now discourage automatic deference to a child's self-declarations on the grounds that the risks outweigh the benefits. They are calling for months-long psychotherapy sessions to address co-occurring mental health problems. Notably, in the United Kingdom, the *Cass Review* attributed the lack of safeguards for children at England's largest pediatric gender center to the "affirmative model," which "originated in the USA."[237]

While American medicine doubles down on invasive and irreversible medical interventions for minors at steadily younger ages, the Old World is restricting transgender treatments for children. Why is Europe so much farther ahead of the US in recognizing the dangers of childhood gender transition? In one sense this has to do with the organization of European healthcare systems: geographically smaller and less populated than the United States, European states tend toward a more centralized pattern. For instance, England had one basic gender clinic, at Tavistock, which became ground zero of the healthy reaction against mutilating gender-confused minors. Of course, centralization is no panacea, as it also makes it easier to impose bad policies upon a population.

Tavistock and the entire medical world were rocked by an internal report by Dr. David Bell, a psychiatrist and staff governor. In 2018, recalls Dr. Bell, "Tavistock Gender Identity Development Service (GIDS) clinicians came to see me as their Staff Governor. They brought concerns about the damage to children as result of the penetration of trans ideology into the [National Health] service. They were too frightened to see me in my room at the Tavistock, emblematic of the climate of fear in organisations which have been ideologically captured."[238]

---

[237] "Independent review of gender identity services for children and young people: Interim report," *The Cass Review*, February 2022, https://cass.independent-review.uk/home/publications/interim-report.

[238] David Bell, "Dr David Bell on the risks to children and young people of a 'conversion practices' ban," CAN-SG, undated, https://can-sg.org/dr-david-bell.

Astoundingly, the number of teenaged girls referred to the Tavistock GIDS had skyrocketed 5,000 percent between 2010 and 2017. And whereas girls had once made up less than 10 percent of gender-dysphoric clients at Tavistock, they now comprised 70 percent.[239]

Dr. Bell took the complainants seriously. After an investigation, he submitted a report to the Tavistock and Portman NHS Foundation Trust that concluded, "the GIDS service as it now functions [is] not fit for purpose and children's ends are being met in a woeful, inadequate manner and some will live on with the damaging consequences." Dr. Bell noted that the Gender Identity Development Service was not taking into account autism, abuse, or other factors that might lead a person to believe he or she is gender dysphoric. Nor did the service appear to have an institutional understanding that gender dysphoria is typically transient—while many of the procedures associated with gender transitioning are permanent.

The Tavistock and Portman NHS Foundation Trust's medical director downplayed the importance of Dr. Bell's investigation, which led to the resignation of psychoanalyst Marcus Evans, one of the trust's governors. In resigning, Evans explained:

> In my 40 years of experience in psychiatry, I have learned that dismissing serious concerns about a service or approach is often driven by a defensive wish to prevent painful examination of an 'overvalued system'.... I do not believe we understand what is going on in this complex area and the need to adopt an attitude which examines things from different points of view is essential. This is difficult in the current environment as the debate and discussion required is continually being

---

239   Janice Turner, "What went wrong at the Tavistock clinic for trans teenagers?" *The Times (London) Magazine*, June 17, 2022.

closed down or effectively described as 'transphobic' or in some way prejudicial.[240]

The whistle, having been blown, echoed far and wide.

The result was the *Cass Review*, which was, to borrow a famous phrase from Thomas Jefferson, a firebell in the night.

Reacting to the Tavistock scandal, the United Kingdom's National Health Service commissioned a policy working group to review the evidence surrounding puberty blockers and hormone treatment for children and young people experiencing gender dysphoria and provide recommendations for clinical care and services. In 2024, after four years of research, British pediatrician Hilary Cass published a nearly four-hundred-page final report which became the largest-ever systematic review of gender-affirming care.

Put simply, this groundbreaking report shattered the foundation of mainstream gender theory.

The final report of the *Cass Review* noted the enormous increase in the number of young people seeking gender-related treatment and the astonishing demographic flip-flop in those asserting gender dysphoria, from prepubescent boys to teenaged girls. These children often carry emotional and mental distresses in a "complex interplay between biological, psychological and social factors." The *Review* also scores "the poor quality of the published studies" on the subject, which tend toward the tendentious.

Dr. Cass's top findings include:

1. There is no way to know which children affected by gender dysphoria will maintain a lasting transgender identity.
2. There is no high-quality evidence for puberty blockers or hormone treatment.

---

240 Jamie Doward, "Governor of Tavistock Foundation quits over damning report into gender identity clinic," *The Guardian*, February 23, 2019.

3. There is no convincing evidence that these medical treatments reduce the risk of suicide in patients suffering gender distress.

4. Children suffering from gender dysphoria should be treated holistically, prioritizing psychotherapy and screening for neuro-developmental and mental health conditions.

On the two critical stages between social transition and surgery, the *Cass Review* emphasizes the attendant uncertainty and murky data and recommends extreme caution. To quote directly:

— The rationale for early puberty suppression remains unclear, with weak evidence regarding the impact on gender dysphoria, mental or psychosocial health. The effect on cognitive and psychosexual development remains unknown.

— The use of masculinising/feminising hormones in those under the age of 18 also presents many unknowns, despite their long-standing use in the adult transgender population. The lack of long-term follow-up data on those commencing treatment at an earlier age means we have inadequate information about the range of outcomes for this group.

In sum, the *Cass Review* calls for putting the brakes on this run-away train:

> For the majority of young people, a medical pathway will not be the best way to manage their gender-related distress. For those young people for whom a medical pathway is clinically indicated, it is not enough to provide this without also addressing wider mental health and/or psychosocially challenging problems.[241]

---

[241] "Final Report," *The Cass Review*, https://cass.independent-review.uk/home/publications/final-report.

Dr. Hilary Cass, namesake and author of the report, was not someone whose opinions could easily be dismissed. She entered this politically charged arena with impressive credentials. Not only was Dr. Cass chair of the Independent Review of Gender Identity Services, but she is past president of the Royal College of Pediatrics and Child Health, past chair of the British Academy of Childhood Disability, and was awarded an Order of the British Empire (OBE) for her services and accomplishments.

She could not be shouted down by shrieks of "transphobe"!

Dr. Cass undertook the project unaware that it would become a landmark of medical literature. "I thought it would be couple of afternoons a month for six months and then I could go home and get on with my retirement," she laughingly told *The Guardian*. Little did she know that it would become "a 24-hour a day obsession" lasting four years.

In conducting the review, Dr. Cass examined fifty studies on puberty blockers and fifty-three on hormone treatments. She found "remarkably weak evidence" in support of their usage. As a result, she recommended "extreme caution" in treating gender-distressed kids. This echoes Do No Harm's calls to review the research behind pediatric gender medicine.

Dr. Cass found that external factors have influenced and stifled conversation around gender identity treatments. For example, she suggests that parents may "unconsciously influence the child's gender expression." Similarly, health professionals are "afraid to openly discuss their views" on these issues due to fear of the social repercussions—or, as we have seen time and again, the termination of their careers.

Dr. Cass's voice is anything but detached and emotionless when she speaks of the human cost of this tragedy:

> We've let them down because the research isn't good enough and we haven't got good data. The toxicity of the debate is perpetuated by adults, and that itself is unfair to the children who are caught in the middle of it. The

children are being used as a football and this is a group
that we should be showing more compassion to.[242]

For years, those with the courage to express trepidation about pediatric gender medicine have had targets placed on their backs. Dr. Cass believes that these attempts to stifle debate not only run counter to the spirit of open scientific inquiry but have endangered kids who might have benefited from public skepticism and debate.

The *Cass Review* rightfully acknowledges that drugs and surgery are not the best way to treat gender-related distress in young people, many of whom will not persist in their feelings of gender dysphoria. Preventing children from accessing these irreversible interventions is the only sensible path forward.

It is absolutely vital that this conversation cross the Atlantic!

Dr. Cass's views are now squarely in the European mainstream. Denmark, Finland, Sweden, Ireland, and Italy have either imposed restrictions on pediatric gender medicine or are currently debating it. That these countries were already taking a more cautious and conservative approach on the treatment of minors claiming gender dysphoria makes the obdurate and intolerant attitude of American gender clinics and clinicians look all the more absurd—and dangerous. As Leor Sapir of the Manhattan Institute observes, the rate of intake-to-medicalization at Denmark's gender clinic fell from 65 percent in 2018 to just 6 percent in 2022.[243]

In Sweden, the esteemed Dr. Christopher Gillberg, professor of child and adolescent psychiatry at the University of Gothenburg and head of the eponymous Gillberg Neuropsychiatry Centre, has called the rush to affirmatively treat trans-identifying children "possibly one of the greatest scandals in medical history."

---

[242] Amelia Gentleman, "'Children are being used as a football': Hilary Cass on her review of gender identity services," *The Guardian*, April 10, 2024.

[243] Sapir, "A Slow Trek Back to Truth?"

Dr. Gillberg deemed the practice of treating these children with puberty blockers and cross-sex hormones "absolutely horrendous." The enormous rush of teenage girls claiming late-onset gender dysphoria includes a disproportionate number of girls with autism or anorexia nervosa, he said. "This identity crisis almost always resolves within a few years," said Dr. Gillberg, who added, "I believe that it is this group that is now recruited by the activists in the field."[244]

Sweden has listened to Dr. Gillberg. Appalled at a ten-year, 1500-percent rise in gender dysphoria among young girls, the Swedes now limit the use of puberty blockers and cross-sex hormones to clinical research settings and in "exceptional" cases. Sweden's National Board of Health and Welfare states children should never receive blockers outside clinical trials, and they must be at least twelve.

As for hormone treatments, a review of eleven of the most progressive Western and Northern European countries (including Sweden) undertaken by Do No Harm's Ian Kingsbury showed that they almost entirely restrict cross-sex hormones until age sixteen, and only upon first undergoing psychotherapy sessions. American children, by contrast, can receive cross-sex hormones at thirteen—and younger in clinical trials.[245]

Finally, every Western and Northern European country we surveyed except one (France) bans "gender-affirming" surgery until age sixteen or, more commonly, eighteen.

By contrast, America has documented cases of minors as young as twelve receiving a voluntary double mastectomy, or what is euphemistically known as "top surgery." What once were isolated and tragic cases are increasingly, and distressingly, common. A study published in the *Annals of Plastic Surgery* revealed that what the authors called "gender-affirming"

---

[244] Jonathon Van Maren, "World-renowned child psychiatrist calls trans treatments 'possibly one of the greatest scandals in medical history,'" *The Bridgehead*, September 25, 2019.

[245] "Reassigned," Do No Harm. See also Stanley Goldfarb and Dr. Miriam Grossman, "Even progressive Europe won't go as far as America in child transgender treatments."

mastectomies "increased 13-fold (3.7–47.7 per 100,000 person-years)" between 2013 and 2020.[246]

While most surgeries on underage youth are double mastectomies for teenage girls, cases of genital surgery—such as the inversion of the penis, sometimes with tissue removed from the colon, to create an orifice resembling a vagina—are documented as well.

Why are children in Stockholm protected from these procedures, yet children in Boston are not?

Though famed for its laissez-faire attitudes toward sexual expression, the Swedes are emphatically rejecting the theory that kids who claim gender dysphoria are suddenly discovering their truer and happier selves.[247]

Meanwhile, the medical establishment in the Land of the Free disgorges such ridiculous claims as that addressing gender distress with psychotherapy instead of blockers, hormones, and surgery is "inflammatory." Incredibly, this article, which appeared in the *New England Journal of Medicine*, suggested legal suppression of "science denialism," which in this case meant dissenting opinions on treatment for gender dysphoria. Censorship and the totalitarian temptation rear their ugly heads in a journal so far gone in wokeism as to border on parody.[248]

This is as pathetic as it is infuriating.

Stifling debate on protecting children is the real affront to science—and a real danger to vulnerable patients. American policymakers would do well to adopt Europe's caution before the country sacrifices any more children on the altar of gender ideology.

---

[246] Annie Tang et al., "Gender-Affirming Mastectomy Trends and Surgical Outcomes in Adolescents," *Annals of Plastic Surgery* 88, no. 4 (May 2022): S325–S331.

[247] Richard Orange, "Teenage transgender row splits Sweden as dysphoria diagnoses soar by 1,500%," *The Guardian*, February 22, 2020.

[248] Meredithe McNamara et al., "Protecting Transgender Health and Challenging Science Denialism in Policy," *New England Journal of Medicine* 387, no. 21 (November 19, 2022): 1919–1921.

- - - - - -

While England and Scandinavia show the way back to some semblance of sanity in halting the transitioning of minors, led by their professional societies, in the United States the professional societies are complicit in these crimes. As with DEI, the permanent bureaucracies within these organizations are pushing much of the change. Their day-to-day management and the lobbyists they employ steer the ship, while the elected boards, which consist primarily of researchers within their fields, keep quiet or mouth the obligatory platitudes, seeking nothing so much as to avoid trouble.

They don't want to upset the apple cart. They serve on the board for a finite period and they have seen what has happened to the few brave men and women who have spoken up against the madness. They are publicly rebuked, even trashed.

Avoiding trouble is a very underrated motivation for inaction.

We would be in a much better place today if, when a parent took a child claiming gender dysphoria to a pediatrician, the doctor said, "Look, we don't know if your child would be better or worse off as an adult if he or she transitioned, so let's begin by sending the child to a psychiatrist to see just what's going on." These simple steps would slow the rush to drugs and surgery and put a stop to much of the madness.

Unfortunately, the pediatrician probably knows that the American Academy of Pediatrics enthusiastically supports transitioning minors. Its policy statement recommends "that youth who identify as TGD [transgender and gender diverse] have access to comprehensive, gender-affirming, and developmentally appropriate health care that is provided in a safe and inclusive clinical space."[249]

Dr. James Cantor, esteemed psychologist and sexologist, has demolished the AAP's pro-transition polemics in the pages of the *Journal of*

---

[249] Rafferty et al., "Ensuring Comprehensive Care and Support for Transgender and Gender-Diverse Children and Adolescents."

Sex & Marital Therapy. This was not a matter of two sides to a debate offering good-faith arguments based in fact and learned opinion. Rather, as Dr. Cantor carefully documents, "the references that AAP cited as the basis of their policy instead outright contradicted that policy, repeatedly endorsing *watchful waiting.*" The AAP haughtily dismissed watchful waiting as "outdated" without explaining why this is so.

The AAP also ignored ten of the eleven then-extant follow-up studies of gender dysphoric children. This was an act of brazen dishonesty, for as Cantor notes, "*every* follow-up study of GD children, without exception, found the same thing: Over puberty, the majority of GD children cease to want to transition."[250]

Lacking entirely a factual foundation, the AAP's policy on transgender and gender-diverse children and adolescents is both dishonest and dangerous. Yet the AAP is seemingly impervious to facts. It is a prisoner of ideology.

Not every medical society acts as a facilitator of child gender transition. In June 2024, the American College of Pediatricians and other dissenting medical organizations signed a Doctors Protecting Children declaration that stated:

> As physicians, together with nurses, psychotherapists and behavioral health clinicians, other health professionals, scientists, researchers, and public health and policy professionals, we have serious concerns about the physical and mental health effects of the current protocols promoted for the care of children and adolescents in the United States who express discomfort with their biological sex.

The American College of Pediatricians and its cosignatories called upon such medical professional organizations as the American Academy

---

[250] James M. Cantor, "Transgender and Gender Diverse Children and Adolescents: Fact-Checking of AAP Policy," *Journal of Sex & Marital Therapy*, 46, no. 4 (2020): 307–313.

of Pediatrics, the Endocrine Society, the Pediatric Endocrine Society, American Medical Association, the American Psychological Association, and the American Academy of Child and Adolescent Psychiatry to "follow the science and their European professional colleagues and **immediately stop** the promotion of social affirmation, puberty blockers, cross-sex hormones and surgeries for children and adolescents who experience distress over their biological sex. Instead, these organizations should recommend comprehensive evaluations and therapies aimed at identifying and addressing underlying psychological co-morbidities and neurodiversity that often predispose to and accompany gender dysphoria. We also encourage the physicians who are members of these professional organizations to contact their leadership and urge them to adhere to the evidence-based research now available [bold in original]."[251]

The AAP's feet need to be held to the fire, as do all professional societies that subordinate the health of children to political and cultural fads—for instance, the Endocrine Society.

The Endocrine Society is a typical subspecialty organization that has been hijacked. It numbers about eighteen thousand and cheerleads "gender-affirming care" for kids.

In June 2023, Do No Harm sent a delegation to an Endocrine Society meeting. One of our people, Dr. Roy Eappen, a distinguished Canadian endocrinologist and unassuming gentleman who happens to be gay, has taken a very forceful public stance against transgender treatment for children. He talked to many of the practitioners at the meeting and found that an extraordinary number of them had no idea whatsoever of what the Endocrine Society was up to—and was pushing,

---

[251] "Doctors Protecting Children Declaration," American College of Pediatricians, https://doctorsprotectingchildren.org. A spokesman for the American Society of Plastic Surgeons, which represents over 90 percent of the plastic surgeons in North America, told *City Journal* that the ASPS "has not endorsed any organization's practice recommendations for the treatment of adolescents with gender dysphoria" and that there is "considerable uncertainty as to the long-term efficacy for the use of chest and genital surgical interventions," given that "the existing evidence base is viewed as low quality/ low certainty." Leor Sapir, "A Consensus No Longer," *City Journal*, August 12, 2024.

in their name. Others "acknowledged that the society's evidence base for pediatric gender transition is weak, at best," said Roy, but "they're afraid to voice their concerns."

As with so many medical organizations, the Endocrine Society is playing to the few, the loud, the activists. Most of its member-practitioners are in the dark, and those who aren't are none too eager to stir up the hornet's nest, for the "society's full-throated endorsement of gender-affirming care implied condemnation of anyone who holds differing views."[252]

When Endocrine Society president Stephen Hammes called Do No Harm purveyors of "misinformation," a group of twenty-one eminent clinicians and researchers from nine countries published a letter in the *Wall Street Journal* disputing the Endocrine Society's position that "gender-affirming" care for minors is salutary. Instead, they said, the preponderance of evidence shows that the risks attendant upon such treatment "are significant and include sterility, lifelong dependence on medication and the anguish of regret." They also noted that gender transition has never been shown to reduce risk and incidence of suicide, and even such a review published by the rabidly pro-transition Endocrine Society concluded, "We could not draw any conclusions about death by suicide."[253]

The letter from these clinicians and researchers was no one-off. The document will be put to excellent use in the legal cases that will go a long way toward determining the future of childhood gender transitioning.

WPATH, the World Professional Association for Transgender Health, styles itself the leading medical organization in all things transgender. Since 1979, when it was known as the Harry Benjamin International Gender Dysphoria Association (it took its current name in 2007), the group has published standards of care that guide many doctors in

---

[252] Roy Eappen and Ian Kingsbury, "The Endocrine Society's Dangerous Transgender Politicization," *Wall Street Journal*, June 28, 2023.

[253] Stephen R. Hammes, "Endocrine Society Responds on Gender-Affirming Care," *Wall Street Journal*, July 4, 2023; Prof. Riittakerttu Kaltiala et al., "Youth Gender Transition Is Pushed Without Evidence," *Wall Street Journal*, July 13, 2023.

their treatment of such patients. But in the winter of 2024, the exposure of its internal communications sent WPATH into a tailspin, for we learned what gender activists say to each other when no one else is around.

Environmental Progress, a think tank led by free-speech activist and Democratic centrist Michael Shellenberger, broke the WPATH scandal with the publication of a 241-page report by Mia Hughes titled *The WPATH Files: Pseudoscientific Surgical and Hormonal Experiments on Children, Adolescents, And Vulnerable Adults.*[254] The report includes screenshots of internal WPATH discussions between 2021 and 2024. Shellenberger introduced this blockbuster with the provocative statement that "these leaked files show overwhelming evidence that the professionals within WPATH know that they are not getting consent from children, adolescents, and vulnerable adults, or their caregivers."[255]

The lawsuits resulting from the WPATH revelations are going to rock their world—and none too soon.

What do gender activists say among themselves?

Most pertinent to the concerns of Do No Harm, WPATH doctors acknowledge that many children who are being transitioned do not comprehend the magnitude of this action. Speaking to the extreme difficulty of getting informed consent from a child for a life-altering procedure, a Canadian endocrinologist lamented to a WPATH Identity Evolution Workshop that he and other gender doctors are "often explaining these sorts of things to people who haven't even had biology in high school yet." A WPATH child psychologist agreed that it is "out of their developmental range sometimes to understand the extent to which some of these medical interventions are impacting them." For instance, "They'll say they understand, but then they'll say something else that makes

---

[254] Mia Hughes, *The WPATH Files: Pseudoscientific Surgical and Hormonal Experiments on Children, Adolescents, And Vulnerable Adults*, Environmental Progress, press release, 2024.

[255] Hughes, *The WPATH Files.*

you think, oh, they didn't really understand that they are going to have facial hair."[256]

Mia Hughes, author of *The WPATH Files*, described some of the ways in which the organization behaved unethically with respect to minors:

> WPATH members believe that minors can understand and give cognitive consent to sex-trait modification interventions that could have a life-long impact on their health, fertility, and future sexual function. In the files, the chief medical officer from Texas advised a concerned therapist to allow a troubled 13-year-old girl to begin testosterone therapy; a therapist discussed starting a 10-year-old girl on puberty blockers; WPATH President [Marci] Bowers openly admitted that natal male children are being left anorgasmic for life; and one surgeon reported performing 20 vaginoplasties on minors.[257]

The aforementioned WPATH Canadian endocrinologist admitted that the lasting consequences of gender-transitioning are lost on some minor patients. "It's always a good theory that you talk about fertility preservation with a 14-year-old," he said, "but I know I'm talking to a blank wall. They'd be like, ew, kids, babies, gross. Or, the usual answer is, 'I'm just going to adopt.' And then you ask them, well, what does that involve? Like, how much does it cost? 'Oh, I thought you just like went to the orphanage, and they gave you a baby.'"

He conceded that some of his long-term patients had expressed if-I-knew-then-what-I-know-now regret: "Now that I follow a lot of kids into their mid-twenties, I'm like, 'Oh, the dog isn't doing it for you, is it?' They're like, 'No, I just found this wonderful partner, and now want kids' and da da da. So I think, you know, it doesn't surprise me." Of

---

[256] Hughes, *The WPATH Files: Pseudoscientific Surgical and Hormonal Experiments on Children, Adolescents, And Vulnerable Adults*, 10–11.
[257] Hughes, *The WPATH Files*, 38. Dr. Bowers, a surgeon, is transgender.

these children, he concedes, "most of the kids are nowhere in any kind of a brain space to really talk about it in a serious way."[258]

It's not as if WPATH was ever a model of disinterested and nonpoliticized scholarship. Dr. Stephen B. Levine, who chaired the committee responsible for the fifth iteration of the "transgender standards of care" in 1998, resigned his position, saying that he had come to the "regretful conclusion that the organization and its recommendations had become dominated by politics and ideology, rather than by scientific process…"[259]

In the most recent revision of its standards of care, WPATH established sixteen as the minimum age for voluntary mastectomies and eighteen as the minimum age for other surgeries, such as penectomies and metoidioplasties. Ignoring legal and ethical boundaries, the Biden administration's assistant secretary for health, Dr. Rachel Levine, intervened, urging WPATH to remove the age recommendations because such limits would add weight to those waging legal challenges to gender surgeries for minors. Unwisely—and significantly—Levine wasn't arguing from a medical standpoint but rather from a purely legal one. The goal was to head off lawsuits, not ensure the best possible care for children.

This story blew up when Levine's relevant emails were released as part of the discovery process in a lawsuit, joined by the US Department of Justice, against an Alabama law banning gender modification. Dr. Levine's chief of staff relayed to WPATH her boss's concern that "specific listings of ages, under 18, will result in devastating legislation for trans care…. She wonders if the specific ages can be taken out and perhaps an adjunct document could be created that is published or distributed in a way that is less visible."[260]

[258] Hughes, *The WPATH Files*, 12-13.
[259] Neal Hardin, "Leaked Files Reveal Ethical Concerns, Pseudoscience in WPATH Standards of Care," Alliance Defending Freedom, April 10, 2024.
[260] Howard Koplowitz, "Biden officials sought to remove gender-affirming care minimum age guideline, Alabama court records show," AL.com, June 25, 2024.

At Do No Harm, we don't care that the erstwhile Dr. Richard Levine now goes by the forename Rachel; that is Levine's business. But by intervening improperly in the revision of the WPATH standards of care, Levine was playing politics with children's health and seeking to provide a legal foundation for the overturning of democratically enacted protections for children.

In response, Do No Harm launched a "Rachel Levine Must Go" petition. We called on Dr. Levine to resign. Failing that, we called on the Biden administration to fire her.

Levine stuck it out. But the Biden White House did back off, issuing a statement that it opposed surgeries for minors, and Levine wound up a featured villain in ads for the victorious 2024 presidential candidate Donald Trump.

Ideally, the trans issue would be dealt with primarily by conscientious doctors, caring parents, and responsible professional organizations. Until that day arrives, Do No Harm is playing a large—the dominant—role in encouraging states to protect children from the trans industry. We hire lawyers to write sound legislation and we hire lobbyists to work with legislators. Our experts testify before legislative committees. Unlike members of Congress, most state legislators are part-time lawmakers. They have minimal staffs, so while many are eager to take on this issue, they lack the capacity to do so effectively. That's where Do No Harm comes in—and does considerable good.

I'm no expert on trans issues, so I leave the expert testimony before state legislative committees to my brilliant Do No Harm associates. We have both a 501(c)3, which is a nonprofit devoted to educating the public and politicians; and a 501(c)4, which is legally permitted to actively advocate for legislation. Donations to the former are tax-deductible; donations to the latter are not.

With the assistance of the Washington, DC, constitutional-liberties law firm Cooper & Kirk PLLC, Do No Harm has designed the Justice for Adolescent and Child Transitioners Act (The JUST FACTS Act).

JUST FACTS prohibits the use of puberty blockers, cross-sex hormones, and surgery to treat an inconsistency between a minor's sex and the minor's perceived gender or perceived sex. It requires school transparency on these issues, prohibits schools from aiding in the transitioning process, limits funding or reimbursement from both public and private sources for these types of treatments, and creates private causes of action for damages for minors who are subjected to treatment that either violates the legislation or causes harm in the future.

As the white paper prepared by Cooper & Kirk (available for free on the Do No Harm website) explains, only a complete prohibition of these treatments will fully protect children and adolescents. We lack high-quality, long-term outcome studies on the causal relationship between hormonal interventions and mental health, and even if such studies existed, it would be impossible to determine with certainty that a particular child or adolescent with gender discordance will persist in that perception. In other words, even if legislation made an exception for "true transgender" minors, it is impossible for clinicians, especially under present conditions, to reliably conclude that a specific minor falls within that category. The cost of misidentifying a minor—that is, prescribing these treatments for a minor whose gender discordance would have resolved on its own—is catastrophic. Thus, only a complete prohibition can fully protect children and adolescents. When a young person turns eighteen, he or she may make his or her own decision.

The JUST FACTS Act addresses the role of schools because there are strong indications that social media and peer pressure have played a substantial part in the dramatic increase of minors who self-identify as having some form of gender discordance. Even non-intrusive interventions at school—like socially transitioning—can make a student's gender discordance worse, thus increasing the likelihood that the student will go on to seek medicalized intervention like puberty blockers and cross-sex hormones. Any solution to this problem must acknowledge the "school-to-clinic pipeline" that feeds the transgender industry.

At present, the JUST FACTS Act is under active consideration in several states. It was passed by the legislature but vetoed by the governor in Kansas, enacted in a slightly different form in Tennessee, and its influence can be seen in the laws passed in Missouri and Utah.

We have a tough fight ahead of us, but we can't help but be flattered when the trans propagandists at *HuffPost* paint us as a nefarious power blocking "trans rights."[261] This is half nonsense; Do No Harm does not oppose the right of adults to transition. Our focus is on protecting children. But we do appreciate *HuffPost*'s recognition of our formidability!

To facilitate justice for young people harmed by the trans industry, Do No Harm has also drawn up a Detransitioner Bill of Rights. It supports those who choose to detransition by protecting five core rights:

— **Informed consent:** No healthcare professional or physician may provide pharmaceutical or surgical treatment to minors to address an inconsistency between the minor's sex and the minor's perceived gender or perceived sex unless the healthcare professional or physician has obtained informed consent from the minor and the minor's parent(s) or legal guardian(s).

— **Effective care:** No city, municipality, or locality may prohibit the provision of mental-health therapy to help a minor address an inconsistency between the minor's sex and the minor's perceived gender or perceived sex.

— **Insurance coverage:** Any gender clinic that uses state funds to directly or indirectly provide or pay for the performance of gender transition procedures must, as a condition of receiving such

---

261 Molly Redden, "A Leonard Leo-linked Group Is Secretly Funding Legislative Attacks on Trans Rights," *HuffPost*, June 24, 2024. See also Jeff McMillan and Kimberly Kruesi, "Meet the influential new player on transgender health bills," Associated Press, May 20, 2023.

funds, agree to provide or pay for the performance of detransition procedures. And any insurance policy that includes coverage for gender transition procedures must also include coverage for detransition procedures.

— **Legal restoration:** State records agencies must develop an expedited process for changing the sex, name, pronouns, and any other information recorded on birth certificates, driver's licenses, or other legal documents for those who detransition.

— **Justice:** Any healthcare professional or physician who provides a minor with a gender transition procedure is strictly and personally liable for all costs associated with subsequent detransition procedures sought by the minor within twenty-five years after the commencement of a gender transition procedure.

At the federal level, Senator Tom Cotton (R-AR) and Representative Jim Banks (R-IN) have introduced the Protecting Minors from Medical Malpractice Act. It makes a medical practitioner who performs a gender-transition procedure on a person under eighteen liable for any physical, psychological, emotional, or physiological harms from the procedure for thirty years after the individual turns eighteen.

And to protect the conscience rights of doctors, nurses, and others, it makes a state ineligible for federal funding from the Department of Health and Human Services if it requires medical practitioners to perform gender-transition procedures against their will.[262]

As I write this in the fall of 2024, twenty-five states have laws, varying in detail, that protect minors against transgender medical interventions. Most of these laws ban surgeries, cross-hormone treatments, or the application of puberty blockers.[263] Several of these laws are currently being contested in state courts.

---

[262] "Protecting Minors from Medical Malpractice Act of 2023," https://www.congress.gov/bill/118th-congress/senate-bill/635.

[263] "States that Protect Minors from Transgender Interventions," Biological Integrity, March 2024, www.biologicalintegrity.org.

For instance, in 2023, the Montana legislature passed and Governor Greg Gianforte signed the Youth Health Protection Act, which bans permanent, life-altering gender-transition medical procedures performed on children. A state district court judge in Missoula issued an injunction blocking execution of the new law, and the matter is now being contested before the Montana State Supreme Court.

The brief filed by Governor Gianforte and various state agencies is worth quoting in part:

> The state of the science on gender-affirming care—nationally and internationally—is currently conflicted and uncertain, and it continues to trend in support of the conclusion that the treatments at issue result in far more harm than good. Yet Plaintiffs claim that children—who cannot vote, purchase alcohol or tobacco, enter into contracts, join the military, or consent to sexual intercourse—can consent to experimental and irreversible procedures likely to exacerbate mental and emotional problems, harm them physically, suppress the natural development of their bodies and brains, and subject them to sterilization.[264]

Montana's Mountain Time Zone neighbor Idaho has also banned gender transitions for minors.[265] Its 2023 law authorizes penalties of up to ten years in prison for physicians who provide puberty blockers, cross-sex hormones, or gender-transitioning surgery to minors.

These laws are just the first steps along our nation's return to medical sanity.

---

[264] "Appellants' Opening Brief," *Scarlet Van Garderen, et al. v. State of Montana, et al.*, February 9, 2024.

[265] "Dr. Stanley Goldfarb Comments on SCOTUS Decision to Uphold Idaho Ban on Gender Transitions for Minors," Do No Harm, April 17, 2024.

- - - - - -

Most physicians I have spoken with—who are generally liberal in politics—are very uncomfortable with the transitioning of minors. The public is stoutly against this; opinion surveys show that 70–80 percent of Americans agree with Do No Harm's position.

As Missouri whistleblower Jamie Reed says, "The doctors I worked alongside at the Transgender Center said frequently about the treatment of our patients: 'We are building the plane while we are flying it.' No one should be a passenger on that kind of aircraft."[266]

It doesn't have to be this way. As an old Dusty Springfield song tells us, all we lack is a bit of courage. Do No Harm and our supporters are supplying that courage.

---

[266]   Reed, "I Thought I Was Saving Trans Kids. Now I'm Blowing the Whistle."

CONCLUSION

BE NOT AFRAID

I ended *Take Two Aspirin* with the exhortation that we all need to stop being afraid.

Are there signs that the fear is abating?

Perhaps—but they are mixed. Anti-Semitism and anti-Israeli sentiment seem to have captured imaginations on campus, though it's impossible to say that this somehow represents an improvement over the DEI cult.

I'm not afraid, but then I'm eighty-one years old. What are they going to do to me? Throw paint on my house? Call me naughty names? I have nothing to lose. Those who do have something to lose—physically, emotionally, and financially—but speak up are the real heroes. They're still in the game yet they refuse to duck into the corner or zip their lip. They challenge the DEI orthodoxy; they speak up for fairness, liberty, and truth. May their numbers multiply manyfold.

Just six weeks before she died in mid-2024, my late friend and inspiration, Dr. Marilyn Singleton, spoke of the need for courage in these challenging times:

Today, advocates for equality and fair, non-discriminatory competition for positions in schools or the workplace hide in another kind of bunker. They shelter in place avoiding the DEI (Diversity, Equity, Inclusion) storm. They are safe from being looked upon by their peers with faux moral revulsion, being labelled a racist or a Neanderthal for not pledging fealty to the 21st Century diversity movement. But their bunker is one of silence, not concrete. And it is only a matter of time before the risk they are avoiding reaches them.[267]

Is this fight winnable? We think so. But even if we can't achieve total victory, we may take heart from the example of Israel. For upwards of seventy-five years it has been surrounded by hostile nations. It has fought wars, it is always on its guard, but it has not only endured but actually gotten stronger.

We just need to keep fighting. To keep educating the citizenry, letting them know what's happening behind the acronyms and happy talk. To keep convincing legislatures and judges and juries that treating people differently because of their race is wrong, and that the chemical and surgical mutilation of confused children is a great evil.

This is a fight worth the battle.

THE END

---

[267] Singleton, "Advocates for Equality Must Emerge from the Bunker and Speak Up."